v4

Heart Attack

DR UNA MACLEAN

Heart Attack

Survival * Recovery * Prevention

GRANADA
London Toronto Sydney New York

Granada Publishing Limited
Frogmore, St Albans, Herts AL2 2NF
and
3 Upper James Street, London WIR 4BP
Suite 405, 4th Floor, 866 United Nations Plaza, New York, NY 10017, USA
117 York Street, Sydney, NSW 2000, Australia
100 Skyway Avenue, Rexdale, Ontario M9W 3A6, Canada
PO Box 84165, Greenside, 2034 Johannesburg, South Africa
61 Beach Road, Auckland, New Zealand

Published by Granada Publishing 1981

Copyright © Dr Una Maclean 1981

ISBN 0 246 11126 7

Printed in Great Britain by
Richard Clay (The Chaucer Press Ltd)
Bungay, Suffolk
Set in Baskerville by
Georgia Origination, Liverpool

All rights reserved. No part of this publication may be
reproduced, stored in a retrieval system, or transmitted,
in any form or by any means, electronic, mechanical,
photocopying, recording or otherwise, without the prior
permission of the publishers.

Granada ®
Granada Publishing ®

Contents

	Introduction	7
1	Is it an emergency?	11
2	Having a heart attack	28
3	A modern epidemic	50
4	Treatment options	70
5	Recovery	86
6	Prevention	108
	A woman's diary	116
	Supplementary reading	137
	Index	140

Introduction

People living in affluent, Western societies are witnessing a virtual epidemic of heart disease. The commonest and most lethal form of this disease is a heart attack. Sometimes it is referred to as 'a coronary' or 'a myocardial infarction'. But no matter how it is named, it is a subject of literally vital importance, especially since most deaths from heart attacks occur within one hour.

This matter is of interest not only to potential victims or people who have already had an attack. It also intimately concerns their families. For instance, although women, through much of their lives, are less likely than men to suffer from this condition, it is usually they who have to cope with a cardiac emergency when it occurs and supervise the patient's recovery, they who are preoccupied with the possibility of another attack and they who agonize over whether there is anything they can do to prevent it happening.

My intention is to provide non-medical readers with an outline of present knowledge and diverging opinions on heart attacks, their contributory causes, what the symptoms are like, the various sorts of treatments and rehabilitative regimes which are currently being recommended from place to place and the conflicting views of doctors about preventive measures.

Reading about how other people have coped with these sudden, deeply disturbing episodes may help those who encounter heart attacks for the first time to take sensible decisions. The latest views of a range of medical experts on the part played by diet, smoking and exercise in affecting liability to a heart attack should aid you in making informed choices between different life styles and their possible effects upon your heart.

The book begins with a series of dramatic accounts from a study I carried out among first-time patients and their close relatives and associates. The events in which they were all unwillingly involved and the complex dilemmas they faced should bring home to you the uncertainty and urgency which still characterize this extremely puzzling disease of our civilization.

My own relationship to the subject matter of this book has changed profoundly since its conception. Originally my interest was purely academic. I knew that cardiologists were critical of what they regarded as patients' stupid delay in calling for medical help when they suffered a heart attack. I thought I should try to find out more about what actually went on in homes and factories when strange, unwelcome symptoms started. What happened during the tense minutes or hours before someone reached for the phone? Did the time that elapsed depend on where the attack occurred, or the time of day or night, or who was present? How did the victims react to the rapidly unfolding drama in which they were suddenly cast in a frightening central role?

I managed to persuade the British Heart Foundation that this topic was worth exploring. Of course it was essential to secure the cooperation of a cardiologist, in this case Professor Michael Oliver, so as to gain access to a series of patients. I was fortunate in having the help of a visiting American social work colleague, Dr Richard Steinman, to interview patients' relatives, and my daughter Aysha Cockshott, then a sociology student, helped in analysing the results of the study.

Little did I think at the time I was collecting my research data that I myself would soon experience the distress attendant upon the diagnosis and treatment of a problematic heart condition. My husband's exceedingly rare and puzzling cardiac illness supervened upon the writing of the research report. His death a year later, from a recurrence of a malignant tumour of the heart, came as I had just signed the contract for this book.

Thus reluctantly caught up in the very doubts, delays and confusions which it was my intention to describe, I found myself virtually paralysed. The difficulty of assuming a proper degree of detachment from a subject which had suddenly assumed intense personal significance at first seemed impossible.

Then I decided that, instead of trying to ignore what had happened, I should turn my own and my family's change of circumstances to the service of a better understanding of the problems of others. That is why I have included extracts from the diary which I kept during my husband's fatal illness.

You must not expect certainties. But I hope to be honest about the impact of heart attacks upon patients, their relatives and society at large and to share my knowledge and experience of how people cope with a mysterious illness of our time.

1

Is it an emergency?

'Is it an emergency?' the doctor's receptionist asked Mrs Campbell, who had phoned as soon as the surgery opened at nine o'clock. The question really put her in a quandary. After all, that was why she had called in the first place, to get help in sorting out her problem, and now she was being asked, in effect, to make a diagnosis herself.

What could she say? It was a matter of comparing the past night with many others just as disturbed but perhaps less disturbing. As the wife of a severely disabled ex-serviceman she was used to dealing with his restlessness and discomfort when his war-wounds were playing up badly. But this time it had seemed different. He had wakened her around 2 a.m., complaining of chest pain, and she had proceeded to ply him with a series of simple remedies. A hot drink, a cheese snack, some Milk of Magnesia were all tried to no avail.

At one point she did wonder whether it might not be a good idea to get medical advice. But they had only recently moved into the district, away from their former GP who was very familiar with his case. And it scarcely seemed justifiable to get any doctor out in the middle of the night.

By breakfast time her nocturnal fears had somewhat

subsided. In spite of continuing discomfort Mr Campbell had at least managed to dress and sit down to the table. His wife's telephoning had been primarily for reassurance; she expected that once they got to the doctor he would prescribe pain killers.

Receptionists are powerful people. Although they are supposed never to refuse an appointment they nevertheless do have to develop their own ways of sorting out people's complaints into those which demand immediate attention and those which can afford to wait. Doctors need this kind of screening to be done for them; they are clear about having to see 'emergencies' at once, so receptionists try to get enough information to put patients in some order of priority, apart from simply 'first come first served'. This time the receptionist was passing the buck back to the patient's advocate, forcing her to say how urgent it was.

At her end of the phone, Mrs Campbell hesitated. She'd got an uncomfortable impression that their last doctor had begun to regard her husband as a bit of a hypochondriac and she didn't want to start off in this practice on the wrong footing.

'Anyway,' she reasoned with herself, 'he's not prostrate, so it can't be an emergency.'

Having reached this conclusion she settled for an afternoon appointment and went to help her husband into the Mini for the morning's shopping expedition.

Returning to the car at one stage she found he was extremely agitated.

'Get me home, get me home,' he pleaded. 'I don't want to die in this car.'

His upper lip was beaded in sweat and his complexion was ashen. No longer in any doubt, she drove him straight to the doctor's surgery and he was referred almost at once to the coronary care unit with the diagnosis of suspected heart attack.

Mrs Campbell's difficulty in sorting out symptoms had been compounded by her husband's long-standing handicaps. Other people had to take into account the fact of recent illness or relatively new complaints which had led them to be already under medical supervision. This was the case with the family of Mr Hardy. He had finally been declared fit to return to his job on the railways after a series of wearisome hospital admissions. The condition which originally took him there had necessitated treatment which led to various 'complications'.

It is estimated that nowadays 12 per cent of illness is 'iatrogenic', that is to say, due to medical treatment. Mr Hardy's family were not clear about the details, but they certainly did not want anything more to do with hospitals. The last of the children had left home and he and his wife had been looking forward to a peaceful period prior to his retirement. On a Saturday morning in June after he had cleaned the car they set out to buy new kitchen equipment for the smaller house they had just been allocated by the local council. But, before visiting the stores, they intended to follow their customary weekend habit and drop in at Mrs Mack's pub, their regular weekend lunch spot.

As he drove there Mr Hardy began to feel acutely ill. He was overcome with such overwhelming weakness that he doubted whether he could manage to get through the traffic lights and find a parking place. He was drenched in sweat, felt a heavy pressure in his chest and wanted to vomit. Negotiating the last block was perilous for everyone near.

Having just made it to the pub he rushed to the toilet

where he was violently sick and had diarrhoea. When he rejoined his wife in the saloon he found himself the focus of female attention. The publican's wife, who knew him well and was a trained nurse, exclaimed, 'He's not at all well, Mrs Hardy, you'd better get him to the Royal.' This was the very place he had just left.

A woman customer, who was a stranger to the pub, nevertheless presumed to add her own gloomy prognostications. 'He looks exactly like my husband when he had his heart attack,' she maintained.

Meanwhile, Mrs Hardy felt strangely dissociated from what was going on around her. It seemed unreal and dreamlike. She could hear the other women discussing her husband and she was aware of his feeble protestations that he would soon be all right. But she could not face the growing transformation of hope into disaster.

As rapid arrangements were set in train for the barman to drive Mr Hardy to the hospital from which he had so recently escaped, Mrs Hardy thought, 'It can't be happening again ... so soon. It's not fair ... '

In their case, there was the added consideration that repeated and protracted absences from work had already endangered his pension rights. So it seemed absolutely essential that he should put in one last, steady period of employment.

Mrs Hardy was temporarily incapable of taking any effective action. She simply rode passively beside her husband on the short trip back to hospital, a most reluctant partner in this cruel turn of fate.

But some women acted very quickly if they were convinced they were facing an emergency.

On a summer Sunday Mr Duncan was dutifully mowing

IS IT AN EMERGENCY?

his parents' lawn when his mother noticed him suddenly crouch down on the grass. She ran out and he muttered something about a terrible pain in his back and the feeling that both his arms had become very heavy. At once she decided that he should go back home, only a couple of blocks away.

As his wife watched him approach she could tell at once there was something seriously wrong.

'My husband is usually a very cheery person,' she told us, 'and you can see it in his face. But this time you could see the pain in his face.'

Nevertheless he put up all sorts of objections when she proposed calling the doctor immediately. First he told her that he knew it was 'only rheumatics'.

'Rheumatics never affect people that way,' Mrs Duncan countered.

'You can't bother the doctor on a Sunday... anyway, I'm not fit to be seen, I'm all dirty, I need a shave,' were his next protests.

Mrs Duncan dealt firmly with all these objections. Ordering him upstairs to wash and change into pyjamas, she reached for the phone, only to be faced with the cold impersonality of a message recorder.

'I'm not one to bother the doctor... but I really think this is an emergency,' she pondered. So she managed to convey an unmistakable sense of urgency in her carefully worded statement.

By the time she ran up to see how he was doing all his initial hesitations had vanished. As he tossed restlessly around, trying to get some relief in the throes of his attack, all that bothered him was the desire for the doctor to arrive quickly.

Another woman, who described her husband as 'a bit of a moaner . . .he complained of the least little thing', was confronted with quite different behaviour when it came to his first heart attack. The severity and suddenness of his symptoms left her in no doubt of their serious nature. She could not possibly confuse this event with his general tendency to fuss. He literally fell to the ground. This time his moans could not be ignored, but it was clear she should not bear them alone.

'I think I was remarkably calm,' she said. 'I'm usually awfully chicken-hearted, but I didn't cry.'

Instead she took a very firm line. Standing over her husband who was writhing on the sitting-room floor she declared, 'I don't care what you say, I'm going to get the doctor and that's that.'

Two days later, as he was being interviewed in the coronary care unit, he confessed to us, 'I've had a thousand warnings and never taken any notice of 'em.' So there had been premonitions of his near disaster. Perhaps it was these early twinges of chest pain about which he had been complaining, always expecting his wife to sympathize but never being prepared to contemplate a medical consultation, since this would have accorded his symptoms a significance he never wished them to merit.

Mr Graham collapsed in the downstairs bathroom. Struggling to his feet he managed to reach the foot of the stairs where he slumped down and began to vomit. His wife's first impulse was to haul him upstairs where he flopped onto the bed, then she rushed down again to phone for the doctor.

In the evening, the family were discussing the day's fateful events in detail. The eldest daughter remonstrated with her mother for having put her father through the ordeal of climbing the stairs.

'But I never knew he'd be going to hospital and I thought bed was the best place for him,' her mother protested.

Later in this book we shall see that an argument is currently raging between doctors in Britain about the matter of home versus hospital treatment, although in other countries hospitalization is still taken for granted. Certainly relatives in these situations are in special difficulties. They not only have to deal with the immediate emergency but they must also envisage its possible outcome. Seeing the manifestations of severe, unfamiliar illness and having little notion of what their doctor may recommend, they simply do the best they can in the circumstances. Few lay people can make a certain diagnosis of heart attack, far less have any conception of arguments among the experts.

Returning to examples of relatives who were puzzled as well as concerned by someone else's suffering, take the case of Miss Doyle, who lived alone with her mother. Roused in the night, Miss Doyle carefully considered her mother's plight and was at first inclined to think she must be exaggerating her pain. A point was reached when her mother asked whether she shouldn't get the doctor to come. Well knowing her mother's dread of hospitals, this allowed Miss Doyle to put her to the test: 'You know that if the doctor comes he may well decide to send you to hospital.'

'Never mind, just call him,' her mother begged, thereby clearly displaying how very ill she felt.

Another nocturnal episode, this time involving a husband and wife, shows the sort of personal clues people utilize in order to interpret the seriousness of a relative's indisposition.

Mr Morris had spent two hours trying in vain to assuage

his wife's pains. He continued to be uncertain of their significance, 'But when she began to tell me where she had hidden the money I knew she was real bad,' he explained to us.

If a person is driven to waken a neighbour this, in itself, is pretty convincing evidence that they are in desperate straits. So when Miss Lawson, a sixty-year-old spinster, struggled across the common landing of the apartment block and managed to rouse her neighbour the latter was already predisposed to concern. Miss Lawson looked both shocked and shocking.

But the sympathetic neighbour hesitated to take the responsibility of calling an ambulance herself because she knew that the sick woman's sister lived near by. So she got her husband out of bed and sent him hurrying off round the block with a second-hand account of what was happening.

After what seemed ages he returned with disappointing news. He had passed on his account to Miss Lawson's married sister who had wakened the doctor. No doubt the tale had lost something of its urgency in repeated telling. At any rate, the doctor's reaction to the story he received by phone was simply to recommend rest. He would be around the next morning, he promised.

When she heard this Miss Lawson's neighbour, who had meanwhile been proffering tea and sympathy, became quite incensed. This was certainly not the outcome she had anticipated when she raised the alarm. So, with the courtesies properly observed, she felt free to take the initiative and summon an ambulance for her distressed neighbour.

Next morning when the doctor turned up on the landing Miss Lawson's neighbour flung open her own door and

IS IT AN EMERGENCY?

shouted triumphantly across at him, 'You'll not find your patient there, she's in the Royal.'

The way she had stage-managed the whole incident obviously gave Miss Lawson's neighbour considerable satisfaction and she recounted the episode with self-righteous gusto.

Several other solitary people had been taken ill at night. One woman 'knocked on the pipes' to attract the attention of neighbours in the next apartment. Another scrambled painfully on hands and knees up the dark tenement stairs, crying out for help. The driver of a morning school bus was on his way to pick up his charges. He turned back at once and painfully drew up at the depot where friends took control of the situation.

Comparative strangers and public servants often acted with alacrity. The detailed circumstances surrounding Mrs Mackay's attack were supplied by the driver of a No. 8 bus.

Mrs Mackay herself recalled that she 'began to feel queer' as she walked to the bus stop near her council house home. But it seemed easiest to board the approaching vehicle and she sank gratefully into a seat. By the time they had reached the general post office her appearance was so unusual that one of the other passengers summoned the driver to take a look at her.

He immediately ordered all the passengers off. Objections were raised.

'They don't like that kind of thing,' the driver explained to us, 'stopping the bus, having to get out and all that. They mutter and mumble and curse about it.'

But he was the man in charge so they had to comply. Soon he managed to enlist a policeman on points duty who backed up his diagnosis of an emergency and called an ambulance.

Mrs Mackay herself had been terribly embarrassed over causing a public scene.

The stage demand for 'a doctor in the house' was a reality in two cases. The first was a Polish housewife who became ill in the street and received first aid in a grocer's shop. The assistants wanted to get her quickly off to hospital but she managed to persuade them that a postgraduate medical student who was her lodger should first attend her. She was accompanied home for this purpose and in fact the doctor recommended her admission, so corroborating the lay opinion.

When a porter in the University Students' Union collapsed the widowed secretary of the club was most solicitous. She suspected that his symptoms were only too like those which had heralded her own husband's death. But the frightened porter felt that Major G, the senior official, should first be told about him. The major domo in his turn called for a 'doctor in the house', in this case a conveniently available final-year medical student. So, when superior authorities are available their judgement is clearly preferred to that of ordinary bystanders.

People on the spot had some strange ideas of what should constitute first aid. When an *émigré* miner from the Ukraine was strolling with friends to the national social club in Edinburgh on a Sunday evening he told them that he had started to have dreadful chest pain. They got him the length of the building and then one of them phoned for an ambulance. But, until it arrived, two of the others frogmarched him up and down in the entrance hall. They seemed determined to 'keep him going', as if they were warding off a collapse by this mechanical means.

Mrs Allison was alone in the kitchen preparing for a big

family lunch when she was taken ill. She had a feeling of great heaviness, she shivered and perspired and felt severe pain across the front of her chest and down her arms. As her husband returned from collecting their son and the grandchildren she flopped into a chair. She looked so very pale and weak that her son was alarmed and hurried immediately to request the use of a nearby phone. But Mrs Allison was determined to go on peeling the potatoes, she was so anxious not so spoil the children's outing. Her husband seemed powerless to help but their neighbour, who had now been made party to the upset, came through from next door. 'That's right,' she said, 'keep working your hands, squeeze your left hand as hard as you can.' Like many heart attack patients, Mrs Allison was complaining of pain in her left arm and hand, so her friend focused on the site of the symptoms. In fact, as we shall see later, this sort of pain is 'referred' from the heart – there is nothing wrong with the arm.

The neighbour also persuaded her friend to walk up and down and tried cold compresses on the back of her neck.

Meanwhile her son was having trouble getting hold of a doctor. He was put through to an exchange when there was no answer from their own GP's surgery. At length he contacted a receptionist who, when she heard him mention 'high blood pressure', agreed to send a doctor along at once. The whole process only took about thirty minutes but seemed much longer to those involved.

Two men were taken ill whilst on the golf course. One of them was Mr Sinclair, whose friend had noticed how his play was deteriorating half-way round. Mr Sinclair, however, at first gave no indication that he was feeling ill and continued until they were nearly at the last hole, where he was finally compelled to sit down.

Such unusual behaviour confirmed his companion's suspicions and he quickly summoned other players to help get Mr Sinclair back to the club-house. Once there, they didn't mention that they were calling an ambulance as they feared it might distress him still further. By the time it came Mr Sinclair was barely conscious. His friend rode with him, supporting his head and anxiously noting his uneasy, rapid breathing as the ambulance sped noisily into town.

So far, most of these true stories have been about people whose symptoms arose suddenly, out of the blue, waking them to a real nightmare or stopping them in their innocent tracks. Admittedly those who were around at the time still had to decide whether they were involved in what doctors might designate a medical emergency. But there was certainly little doubt that something quite unusual and disturbing was afoot and the questions resolved themselves into how, and how quickly, a doctor should be called or whether, in fact, it would be better to get hold of an ambulance directly.

But one big problem is that by no means all heart attacks are equally dramatic and it is when an illness is gradual or intermittent that everyone, including the doctor, has considerably more difficulty in deciding about or diagnosing it. This difficulty is compounded if the patient is alone at the outset.

An elderly widower had been suffering for a week from what he regarded as 'chest trouble'. One Sunday morning he felt so much worse that he stayed in bed. By now he had decided that it must be indigestion and he fervently hoped it would ease off. Instead, in spite of everything he tried, his pain got steadily worse so that, by noon, he was forced to shout for help.

His calls were heard by the middle-aged spinster next door. But she chose at first to ignore them, feeling that she might be compromised if anyone saw her going alone into a single man's house. Eventually she resolved her dilemma over respectable appearances by shouting to a neighbouring couple opposite them who proceeded to force their way in through the old man's back door.

Another man's general practitioner had first seen him very soon after he developed suspicious chest symptoms. The doctor had diagnosed angina and confined him to bed, as a precautionary measure. When the weekend was over Mr Anderson's wife was in a special quandary because his illness was so poorly defined, its seriousness apparently uncertain even in the careful doctor's estimation. She had a job, which was all the more necessary to them during his indisposition. Whilst she could not afford casual absences she would naturally be prepared to stay off, and justify so doing, if she could be sure her husband was seriously ill.

She reasoned with herself thus: 'He is doing all right and if I stay at home he will worry and think he is worse than he is.' So off she went. Shortly after she had gone her husband's pains became much more severe. Of course we cannot be sure that they did not feel worse to him once he was left totally alone. Perhaps her absence was more alarming than her presence would have been.

He got out of bed, made his way down thirteen stairs and phoned to tell the doctor that the pains were worse. An ambulance was sent to take him direct to hospital. When Mrs Anderson heard about this dreaded dénouement she was stricken with remorse, feeling she had made the wrong decision. Immediately she planned to install a telephone extension in the bedroom. 'I'd feel terribly guilty if it happened again and he couldn't reach the phone,' she explained to us when he was clearly on the mend a few days later.

A solitary seaman on leave was peacefully trimming his hedge when he was assailed by severe chest pain and vomiting. He resolved at once to go round to his sister's place. But long service training had made him reluctant to appear dishevelled in public, so he struggled to 'wash and dress immaculately', in the words of his sister.

In spite of his efforts to maintain superficial appearances she was appalled by how he looked when he turned up on her doorstep. Her first impulse was to rush off and make up a bed for him. The prospect of hospitalization did not occur to her. 'I'll have to change the sheets if he's going to be sick in my house,' she thought, seeing herself as his natural nurse and helper.

Not every woman relative was so sympathetic, however. When Mr O'Brien got home late on Saturday night from the miners' club and proceeded to thrash about in the bedroom, complaining volubly, his wife concluded that he was simply 'drunk again'. So she turned her back upon his groans and pleas and could only be persuaded to take his condition seriously when dawn broke.

We spoke to her and her mother together shortly afterwards and they were united in their conviction that the victim's heart attack was a sign of divine retribution.

'God's slow but He's sure and He got him in the end,' declared his mother-in-law, with obvious satisfaction.

'He was a right mean man. He never took any notice of me when I was ill and he'd never give the kids a penny,' his wife added.

IS IT AN EMERGENCY?

For his part, Mr O'Brien was duly depressed by his fate. In his solitary bed in the intensive care unit he told us how much he hated to sleep alone. He was really missing his wife.

At times a series of friends, relatives and strangers might be involved at the start of a heart attack.

Mr Renton worked in a large electronics factory which boasted a first-aid room complete with a trained nurse. On the morning of the day in question he started to feel faint and confided in his workmate on the bench. 'I think I may be having a bit of a heart attack,' were his words, after which he never once repeated his deepest fears.

His mate suggested he should consult the nurse. But he put off doing so until after he had tried to eat his fish and chips lunch. When he did see her she was unimpressed by his symptoms. Returning home, he was judged by his wife to be far from well. She very much wanted him to go round to the doctor's evening surgery. But Mr Renton stoutly maintained that it was nothing more serious than a stomach upset.

The afternoon wore on in fruitless argument. Presently the 'insurance lady' turned up to collect the weekly premium.

'What's the matter with him, then?' this regular visitor enquired.

'He's a terrible man, he's not feelin' well but he won't let me get the doctor to him,' Mrs Renton explained.

'It's just the fish, just the fish I had at lunch,' Mr Renton interjected.

'How many other people felt sick at the plant?' the lay diagnostician shrewdly enquired.

'None that I know of,' said Mr Renton sheepishly.

At this the 'insurance lady' imperiously declared, 'Don't play around, Mrs Renton, I don't like the sound of it, get the doctor at once.' And the unwilling victim had to comply.

For a relative on his or her own, dealing with a recalcitrant patient can prove very awkward and require careful strategies.

Mr Jones was a retired bank manager whose doctor had been treating him for anginal chest pains over several years. Experiencing a bout of much more severe pain one morning he promptly reacted by preparing for a long walk with the dog, just to prove to himself his heart was all right.

'Angina's angina and that's all there is to it,' he told his anxious wife, dismissing her fears with irrefutable logic. On his return she could see he was still unwell but at first felt powerless to change the situation.

As night fell the domestic pet featured once again in this suburban drama. This time it was Mrs Jones who sallied forth, on the pretext of walking the terrier but in fact going straight to phone the doctor from the nearest public call box.

When their medical adviser 'happened to drop in' shortly afterwards Mr Jones resisted the suggestion that an ambulance should take him to hospital. Instead, consistently in control, he himself summoned a taxi.

People often try hard to act normally and responsibly in the face of increasing discomfort. Early one morning the boiler-man at the Dental Hospital was seen to stagger and hold his hand to his chest.

'Did you take a bad turn?' one of the cleaners asked, and he told her she had better phone for a doctor. But, while they were waiting for an ambulance to come, the alarm bell rang from the boiler, indicating that the pressure was rising to a dangerous level. The boiler-man said he must go down and tend the boiler and he refused to let his workmate, Mrs Tait, take instructions instead.

'He's a worker,' she attested as she described how he had dragged himself downstairs, closely followed by her in case he collapsed.

One man didn't mention his increasing pain to his wife as they were preparing to visit friends. Only towards the end of the evening did she notice how unwell he looked. She was moved afterwards by what she told us must have been his motives. 'He didn't want me to know because he knew I wouldn't have let him go out and he didn't want to disappoint me.'

2

Having a heart attack

The incidents narrated in the last chapter are the sort that doctors would probably have called emergencies but which presented untutored lay people with considerable problems to begin with. After the event it is easy to be wise but the beginnings of things are very puzzling.

Heart attacks are characteristically sudden events and carry a real risk of death. So it is important to discover whether any avoidable delay occurs in getting someone within reach of expert advice and attention. I carried out a survey in Edinburgh in the summer of 1975, amongst a group of seventy-seven consecutive patients who had recently been admitted to a coronary care unit. None of them had ever had a heart attack before and so they and their associates were faced with a new experience. We were concentrating on what they told us had occurred before a doctor or an ambulance had been called.

All the patients were interviewed in hospital, usually within forty-eight hours of admission. This meant that most of them were seen in the coronary care unit before they were considered to be past the acute danger period and ready for transfer to another ward within the hospital.

HAVING A HEART ATTACK

The decision to obtain expert help must have been made by a non-medically qualified person, either the patient or someone else upon the scene at the time, so we were not interested in those whose heart attack had developed whilst they were already patients in this or any other hospital.

Frankly, the people we describe cannot be regarded as completely typical cases of heart attack within the Edinburgh community at this time. Those we met were the lucky ones, the survivors. We know nothing at all of the circumstances surrounding the sudden deaths of those unfortunates who died without the benefit of any hospital attention, nor do we have information relating to patients treated at home.

Although we know from other evidence that it is possible to survive a heart attack without ever being medically diagnosed, from our vantage point we could clearly never discover any of these cases. Finally, the individuals we saw in the unit were not all residents of Edinburgh; some had come in from towns and villages near by.

Supposing one were to design an ideal piece of research into people's reactions as a heart attack developed, what would it entail? Ideally one would need to be around with them for the entire time as they went through the whole process. Memories are short and we are all continually engaged in reconstructing our past in the light of our present. So what someone recalls and recounts may be inaccurate and incomplete. Especially, if patients are asked in a hospital ward by a researcher whom they know to be a doctor, they may modify their statements in one way or another, saying what they think you would like to hear.

But it is clearly out of the question to research this subject any other way than by asking people after the event, for the obvious reason that no one knows who is fated to have a heart attack. Moreover, our entire life as well as the work of every doctor is based upon using people's everyday accounts of what has happened to them. So we are here in fact considering seventy-seven case histories.

But we did not confine our interest to what the patients had to tell us. In the great majority of instances they had been incapacitated by the attack and reliant on others to act on their behalf. It was essential, therefore, to seek out all the witnesses, helpers, relatives and workmates we could find to supply their supplementary accounts of what had transpired and enable us to build up a multi-dimensional picture.

These associates of the patient were identified as soon as possible after someone was admitted to the unit. Finding them was rather like a detective operation at times. We had to track down golfing companions, mates in a work gang, policemen and employers, not to mention the numerous relatives who formed the bulk of the patients' associates.

Most of them were seen outside the hospital setting, in their own homes or places of work. There was plenty of time to go into detail with them; they were not wearied by illness and often had a great desire to 'tell it how it was'.

We did try to complete an interview with every patient on the list, but in a few cases this was not possible or humane and we had to renounce the attempt or be content with a shortened account, concentrating on key items.

As far as the patients' friends and relations were concerned, they were usually very cooperative once they were tracked down. But we did not venture to intrude upon the grief of the relatives of a few patients who died in hospital. And one woman heart attack victim explained to us that she did not want her husband to be bothered with questions. Until her sudden collapse she had been caring for him, alone at home, where he was dying of cancer.

First I shall summarize some basic facts about these heart attack patients. Fifty-five out of the seventy-seven were men. Almost 90 per cent of the entire group fell between the ages of forty-five and sixty-nine but there were two below the age of forty and two over seventy. Sixty-two patients were married. Half had never gone beyond the stage of primary education. Twenty-three people lived in their own houses, rather more occupied public housing, rented from the local council.

Over two-thirds knew someone who had had a heart attack. This kind of first-hand knowledge was the main source of ideas and opinions about heart disease, but eleven mentioned TV programmes and the same number mentioned newspapers.

It was exceptional for anyone to say that there had been a marked change in their home circumstances or at work. In other words, we did not uncover evidence of special sources of distress or stress which some suspect as triggering attacks.

We asked everyone to try to describe what their general health had been like in the period before the episode which landed them in hospital. Almost 38 per cent told us they regarded their health as 'good' beforehand, only 32 per cent considered they had been in poor health.

All the same, it was interesting that nearly half the patients told us that they had seen their own GP during the previous four weeks. Only a few had consulted on account of new symptoms; in most cases it had been because of some longstanding medical problem. However, twelve had had an electro-cardiogram (ECG, an electrical test of the heart muscle) at some time in their lives.

A third of those we talked with said they had felt unusually tired or lethargic of late. The same proportion noted, in retrospect, how they had been cutting down on non-essential tasks, sometimes formerly agreeable activities like visiting the library or organizing a record collection, in other cases weekly cleaning or sorting laundry.

Probing into the symptoms and sensations they experienced just before admission, we were trying to discover how they distinguished their recent troubles from what had been a previously normal state of health or, at least, only moderate disability.

Pain or discomfort in the front of the chest was by far the commonest first symptom. People described it as a sensation of heaviness or pressure and often said it had felt as though a firm band was being drawn tight around them.

By the time help was summoned the initial symptom had usually been accompanied by a whole set of other alarms and discomforts. For example, thirty-five people had broken out into a cold sweat, thirty-eight experienced pain in the arms, shoulders or neck; eighteen were very restless; twenty-one felt extreme anxiety. Breathlessness (without any cough), vomiting and a sense of faintness or blurred consciousness were experienced by many.

At the time 'the attack' (as they subsequently regarded it) began forty of the patients (62 per cent) had been at home, fifteen were at work and the rest were engaged in some leisure pursuit or travelling.

Sixteen patients were alone when their symptoms started and we gave examples in the last chapter of how some of them coped. The commonest situation, however, was for one of the family to have been present. Nearly all the rest had friends, workmates or a neighbour near.

Patients had attributed all sorts of causes to the initial symptoms, the commonest being indigestion. Nineteen declared that it had never crossed their minds that they might be having a heart attack. But thirteen did admit to an early suspicion that this might be the case, and twenty were driven more strongly to this conclusion as the symptoms grew worse.

A third of the patients described how the initial symptoms had rapidly worsened, over the course of fifteen to thirty minutes. In another third the process took from half an hour to one and a half hours. We saw earlier what transpired in a number of such cases. Here are several more.

Mr Richards, a civil servant, aged thirty-eight, was the youngest person in our entire series. Within three-quarters of an hour of first feeling chest pain and weakness he had taken himself by taxi to the Accident and Emergency Department of the hospital. His whole process of self-diagnosis was remarkably quick and accurate. Possibly the way he responded to his symptoms was not unconnected with the fact that both his father and his brother had died of 'coronaries'.

Mr Hearst was out ploughing when he felt a dreadful tightness in his chest. He thought at once it might be a heart attack and told the farm manager who commandeered first a tractor then a van to get him quickly back home. The van waited outside the cottage to run Mrs Hearst up to the farm phone. But she thought, 'I just couldn't leave a man with a heart attack sitting in the kitchen chair looking so blue and cold.' So she helped him into bed first.

No one was in any doubt about the seriousness of his condition and the fact that this part of the process took an hour and a half was largely due to the distances involved. As it happened, their doctor was out, but the receptionist guaranteed to contact him on his rounds within twenty minutes. Afterwards came the ordeal of a twenty-mile ambulance journey to the city hospital.

Mr Patterson was head barman in a village pub. He told us afterwards that he did have what he considered a bout of indigestion on Tuesday night, but he didn't mention it to his wife and went off in good spirits to work the next morning. As soon as he reached there, at nine o'clock, his chest and left shoulder became extremely sore and he felt giddy. We got the rest of the story from his wife and daughter and an early chance customer at the inn.

It was indeed fortunate that this man had dropped in for he was a witness to Mr Patterson's sudden restlessness, his going outside for a breath of air, the way he loosened his tie, and eventually lay down with 'a faraway sort of glazed look'. On Mr Patterson's own request, the concerned customer drove quickly off for his wife. She was very distressed by his appearance and phoned the doctor at once before covering her husband gently with her coat and trying to cushion his head on the customer's folded jacket.

She told us later how he had been very irritable in the previous few weeks, shouting at the children in a quite uncharacteristic fashion and complaining about having their companions about the house. She had noticed several other changes in his behaviour. He had stopped several times while doing the garden ten days before, saying half seriously that he must be getting old, and wondering about the state of 'his old ticker'. Whenever he was resting indoors she saw he had got in the habit of rubbing his left arm and clenching and unclenching his hand. He usually took a brief afternoon nap between shifts but lately the family would have to shake him awake after two hours. He did consult his doctor not long before his attack but never mentioned his arm trouble,

HAVING A HEART ATTACK

requesting help instead for something entirely different.

Returning to the way symptoms developed for most people, a third did not have the steady, remorseless increase of chest pain which was such a feature of the majority. Instead, they reported having experienced more confusing, fluctuating sensations which came and went over an extended period of time.

In part this may be due to the differing tolerance of individuals to pains and discomforts. But it could also be that people were editing their personal history for us, including in some cases early feelings of unease as part of what later evolved into the full-blown attack and, in other cases, separating the dramatic, final event in their own minds from the assorted premonitory pains and discomforts of previous days.

Mr Newsam, who worked in a brewery, admitted once he was in hospital that he had begun to have chest pains when out with his wife the evening before admission. But he told no one and got up at 4.30 as usual for the early shift. Getting there involved a 1½-mile walk and he found he had to stop several times on the way until the pains eased off. He said to his mates he felt 'awful woozy – pains in my chest'. This went on all morning and so he tried to get through to his doctor on the phone. When he did make contact, around noon, he was told he could either be seen in ten minutes at the surgery or return in the evening.

The first alternative seemed a clear impossibility to Mr Newsam who would never have contemplated calling a taxi for himself. So he left the brewery and made his way painfully home by bus. Happening to glimpse him as he neared the door his wife was startled to realize he must be ill. She wanted to summon the doctor but he wouldn't hear of it in view of the promised evening appointment, and their married son who dropped in also tried in vain to get him to change his mind. As he and his wife eventually made their way to the doctor's by public transport he refused to take his pyjamas with him, putting out of his mind any possibility of hospitalization.

When one of his workmates called in a few days later to enquire after his progress Mrs Newsam remonstrated with him over the way the chaps at work hadn't hustled her husband to the doctor. His friend replied, 'Och, missus, we can't be running to the doctor every time we get a wee pain like some of those so-and-so's down here.'

Mr Smith, a 54-year-old mechanic, was troubled with chest pains, which he took to be indigestion, over the course of two days and felt excessively tired. By Monday evening the pain became 'terrific', he lay on the settee thumping his chest. All the same he insisted that he did not need a doctor and his wife reckoned her best policy was to let him have his way. Next morning he rose with a struggle. During that same afternoon, he capitulated, saw his doctor and then drove himself to the Royal Infirmary.

It turned out that over half of the patients had outside help very quickly summoned for them, in less than one hour. Twenty-five people took between one and twelve hours and five had endured for over four days. The most striking difference was between those who took under or over one hour to summon assistance. Shortly we shall see what general factors were associated with longer or shorter times before summoning help. It is however abundantly clear that, although there may be arguments, most people do not waste time once severe symptoms are present.

We imagined that perhaps the availability of a telephone

might be crucial. But there proved to be no problem in locating phones and getting permission to use them in crises like these.

The person who is actually going through a heart attack generally reaches a point when he is compelled to tell others about his pain. But the people who are around at the time use many other indicators of the nature of the illness, taking into account what they know or have lately noticed about the sufferer. According to Irving Zola, an American sociologist: 'Virtually every day of our lives we are subjected to a vast array of discomforts. Only an infinitesimal amount of these get to the physician. Neither the presence nor the obviousness of the symptoms, neither the medical seriousness nor the objective discomfort seem to differentiate the episodes which do and do not get professional treatment. So what does convert a person to a patient?'

Zola claimed that the eventual decision to seek medical help was often reached because of some change in the interpersonal relationships in which the individual was involved. Alternatively certain people would only countenance involving outside aid once such a course of action had been approved or recommended by others.

He was mainly considering the process of becoming a patient as it was experienced by people with slowly developing, progressive disorders. But the possibility of accommodating to a variety of warning symptoms, even if chest pain constituted one feature of the picture, does come into this.

In the patient with a coronary the move to seek help is necessarily speeded up. The average period from the start of more severe chest pains turned out to be only 1½ hours. Undoubtedly, during this pre-hospital period, we met many examples of the doctor being called because of pressure from someone else. In fact, the patient was often inevitably passive. But in numerous cases the victims themselves, though in considerable pain, kept trying to avoid being regarded as patients by others, for instance by withholding early symptoms or not admitting the increasing severity of their pain.

How did the patients' associates deal with the diagnostic problems which they unexpectedly faced?

It is mainly men who have heart attacks and women who must cope. Forty-eight of the seventy-seven patients' associates whom we interviewed were women. Rather younger than the men, on the whole, mostly wives, some daughters. As well as talking to close relatives and friends, we listened to the tales of bystanders and workmates.

They reported knowledge about heart attacks from many different sources – for example over 80 per cent knew someone who had suffered one. By discussion with others many people had constructed some sort of picture of what it might be like. Indeed nine said they had experienced the condition themselves.

Naturally wives and husbands were in the best position to comment on any recent changes in the patient's activities. The commonest observation had been of someone seeming overtired. Others had seemed unusually irritable, slowed down in their walking or letting things slide. Some people had been neglecting common household chores, or had been devoting less attention than usual to other members of the family. Thirty-five of the associates noticed that the patient had been more inclined to take naps.

Most people had reached their own conclusions about the nature and onset of symptoms, more than half had been

HAVING A HEART ATTACK

impressed with the suddenness of the attack.

As might be expected, people went into a great deal of detail when it came to describing the appearance and behaviour of the victim in the throes of the attack, a very traumatic time for all concerned. They reported on the patients' cries of pain, their breathlessness, sweating and restlessness, their desperate twisting and turning in the attempt to find relief, their vomiting, their staggering and stumbling with dimming consciousness to complete collapse.

Those who were present had been especially struck by the changes in someone's facial appearance which had presaged or accompanied an attack. Only eight people had noticed no change in the victim's complexion; the rest remarked on how very pale or grey or even green he or she had looked. A cold sweat had seemed a particularly alarming accompaniment of an attack, very probably because of the association with the chill of death.

People were asked to give their judgments on what they regarded as predominant traits in the patients' personality. Over 70 per cent of the associates, nearly all wives, described them as 'stubborn'. Another very common appraisal of the male patient was 'someone who wouldn't give in to defeat'.

Faced with this crisis, usually in the home, the patients' associates did what seemed best in the circumstances. Usually they aimed to get the patient into bed. One wife consulted a home doctor manual. 'I put him in "the semiprone position", like the book said', she told us, 'but he was soon out of bed again and rolling about on the floor.'

It was striking how often patients were picked up or dragged off the floor and forced to climb the stairs in the direction of the bedroom. Of course a proportion (21 per cent) of attacks began in bed, at night. But women were frequently very concerned to settle someone who was so clearly ill in 'the best place for him, bed'. This often necessitated changing into pyjamas and several had their hands and faces washed. Sometimes this procedure was a prelude to an anticipated home call by the doctor, otherwise it was simply part of appropriate home care.

There was a clear tendency for delay in summoning outside help to be greatest if the patient was at home in bed, although patients who were wakened by pain usually did tell someone else very quickly. By contrast, expert help was rapidly called if they were at some place of leisure or entertainment. It was not, however, the case that delays were minimized at work.

It may be that someone in bed already feels reasonably secure. Or else he may have learnt, over time, that troubles which loom large during the night seem less dreadful in the clear light of day. There is also an added seriousness attached to summoning a doctor out at night – it is an admission by the caller that he and his relatives have defined the situation as a real emergency.

The relatively long delay at work was unexpected. But some patients, especially men, were very reluctant to evince weakness at work, in front of workmates. They tried to hide their early symptoms and determined to carry on, at least until they could get home where they expected to receive womanly care and sympathy.

At a place of leisure or in some other public place the victim of a heart attack is likely to be among a group of comparative strangers. Anything in the nature of a collapse will galvanize others into action. They do not want to be charged with negligence.

'I called the ambulance right away,' one club manager told us. 'After all, I didn't want to be left with a death on my hands.'

Moreover, someone obviously incapacitated constitutes a peculiarly incongruous element in what is supposed to be a place of enjoyment and relaxation. It is definitely not good for business.

In the comfort and privacy of home it is possible to slide gradually and easily into illness. One can subside into a chair, stretch out on the couch or 'just go into the bedroom for a bit of a lie down'. There are places to be off colour, the bathroom is convenient, simple remedies for pain and discomfort are available in the medicine cabinet and on the kitchen shelves. Warmth, a hot drink, alcohol, antacids and previously prescribed medicines are all close at hand, ready to be supplied by relatives who hasten to dispense sympathetic aid.

Patients who had had occasion to visit their doctor during the previous month were significantly less likely to call him during an attack than those who were not currently under medical care. Partly this is a measure of the suddenness of some attacks. But, on the other hand, patients already on medication may have felt that their health was being adequately monitored. In some cases the actual symptoms of chest pain which eventually led to a call for help were being treated as angina, and several people reported how they reached for their pills in the expectation that they would work this time as formerly. Where symptoms had been present off and on for a time they were certainly normalized by some patients, taken for granted and not perceived as anything liable to get worse.

This came out in regard to patients whose friends and

relations had noticed they had become increasingly irritable. There was a tendency when this had been the case for more time to elapse before getting help. Here perhaps the patients' associates had become accustomed to a series of minor complaints. Quite frequently, in the latter portion of our interviews with them, they would remark how they had never realized until after the event the way in which the illness they were now describing had actually been building up over a considerable period of time.

This might come to be seen, from the relatives' point of view, as a tendency for the patient to neglect his own health. Apparently negligence over symptoms seemed to be defined as reluctance to tell one's doctor about them as opposed to sharing them with the family. We shall be returning to the whole subject of reluctance or resistance to seeking medical help later in this book.

At this point another key finding is important. When the person with the patient was a woman the period between the onset of an attack and the call for specialist help seems to have been longer. A spouse or child of the patient was associated with a significantly longer delay time. How do we account for this?

In the first place there is the matter of differences in the customary roles of the sexes. Many of the women associates were wives, daughters or other female relatives, accustomed to performing a protective, nurturing role. Looking after the patient as best they could, providing 'tender, loving care', they were in effect substituting for professional medical assistance which was only to be utilized as a last resource.

It was also clear that a number of wives found it difficult to change quickly from a position in which they had been accustomed to let their husband rule the household and make the key decisions to one in which the situation was reversed. Suddenly a woman was faced with going directly against a man's wishes, defining him as weak and helpless, and calling upon another man to confirm his humiliating dependence. Some time may have to elapse or, at least, certain negotiations must be undertaken, before someone who is used to thinking of himself as strong and dependable can be prevailed upon to renounce this whole self-image.

We found that the presence of a woman was associated with increased delay time, even if the patient was not specifically objecting to medical help being called. But, if the patient's associate was a man, they were more inclined to defer to the victim's own preferences.

A number of the men in these settings were workmates, some were strangers, a few were golfing companions. To the extent that these tended to be secondary relationships, rather than the intimate family relationships which usually held when the person closely involved was a woman, the men present might well be more respectful of the patient's expressed wishes. Such circumspection could lead to minimum delay when the patient did not resist medical help but rather longer delay when someone was able to make their objections to such assistance quite explicit.

By far the most important factors determining how soon people sought for help were the mode of onset of the symptoms and their intensification. The more suddenly the attack occurred and the faster symptoms seemed to be intensifying the more rapidly help was sought.

The source from which help was sought also came into the picture. Thus, a call could have gone directly to a doctor; it might, more often, have been mediated through a secretary or a receptionist; the call could have been made to the ambulance centre or the police (by dialling 999); in two instances the patient drove or was driven to hospital with no agent intervening.

There had clearly been an atmosphere of intense haste and alarm when people decided to call directly for an ambulance. Conversely, making contact with the GP through a receptionist seemed to have been indicative of a more problematic situation, where the people on the spot couldn't be sure if it was an emergency but they did want the doctor to come and sort it out for them and dispense more powerful treatment than they could provide unaided. If people were quite certain of their own diagnosis and determined to get someone to hospital they could not bear to wait for a doctor to arrive.

Another way of looking at this is to consider the mode of transport to hospital. Nearly two-thirds of those who were brought in by an ambulance, which was summoned by the doctor once he reached the house or after he had examined the patient in his surgery, took over an hour to involve the doctor in the first place. But more than 80 per cent of those who summoned an ambulance directly called it themselves (or their associates did) in less than an hour. For a few cases, at the outset of this study, the mobile coronary care ambulance was available. It was called fastest, clearly indicating a confident and precise diagnosis on the part of the caller. The decision to involve the local doctor as the first line of expert help was an indication of less urgency or more uncertainty.

We found that in numerous cases the victims themselves, though in very considerable pain, would persist in trying to avoid being defined as a 'patient' by others, by withholding symptoms from those around them, denying their severity or playing down their possible significance. 'He knew if he told me just how he felt, I'd insist on the doctor,' as one wife said.

Some patients spoke graphically of the fear of impending death which had accompanied the attack.

'I felt as if doom was about to strike me,' one woman remembered. 'I thought I was away,' were the words two men used.

No doubt many felt in mortal danger and were desperately trying to reassure themselves. But, even if they did not realize their condition could be fatal, a large number of them specifically feared being sent to hospital. As their strength ebbed from them they still tried to delay a move from their normal, secure setting to a place where they would have to submit without question to medical orders.

We came upon several cases where relatives spoke of this, for example, 'She tended to keep symptoms to herself, she had an extreme fear of hospital.' Others, like Mrs Donald, spoke of her husband's attitude as 'He's an awfu' man for doctors.'

We said earlier that people may have become gradually used to an accumulation of symptoms building up over days or weeks. But we also had plenty of evidence that withholding information about symptoms or their severity was frequently happening. It was an important way of preserving someone's self-image as a strong, healthy individual, a person who may be suffering but who will stoically endure and try to make light of it.

Patients who had withheld symptoms might boast about it later on in hospital, thus gaining justification for the need to be admitted to an intensive care unit whilst at the same time enhancing their reputation for courage by having held out for so long.

The importance to some men of concealing symptoms to promote a masculine image was made quite explicit by Mrs Grant who said, 'He's always held back his symptoms, mainly because he felt it a sign of weakness or unmanliness to complain.' A lot of relatives told us that this kind of concealment was normal. Mrs Norman said, 'He rarely complains, you've just got to notice he's not right.' Another told us, 'He wouldn't mention discomfort at all but if he was in pain he'd describe it as discomfort.' People like these are therefore taken very seriously the minute they did complain.

Similarly, when patients whose relatives knew they normally resisted medical treatment conceded that a doctor was necessary or actually demanded that the GP be called, those relatives were automatically impressed by the gravity of the situation. Then there were others, like Mr Jordan, for whom to report any early discomforts would have threatened his claim to 'particularly good health...never had a day's illness in my life'. It was important for him that this illness should be known to be sudden and severe.

We had to look very closely at our data to discover just how many had been withholding symptoms even as the severe chest pains of the attack were assailing them. Twelve out of sixty-five had behaved this way. They included patients who summoned medical help themselves without any prior discussion with others, patients who admitted withholding symptoms during the attack and also patients who refrained from wakening their spouse when the attack began.

But this sort of information was not necessarily given to me, when I interviewed patients in hospital; it often had to be inferred from what they confessed to others. This was scarcely surprising in view of the nature of a hospital interview. The patient has to make sense of the questions he or she is being asked and will also try to guess what the investigator is likely to regard as proper answers.

The interviewer was a doctor, patients were in bed in an intensive care unit, tied down by monitoring leads, surrounded by medical experts and acutely aware of the life-threatening experience they had just been through. Possibly they were feeling some guilt about not seeking expert care sooner. They might well feel it inappropriate, in such a high-powered medicalized environment, to tell a doctor they had been so irresponsible as to conceal symptoms. We came across a specific example. Mrs Poole never revealed to the cardiologist that she had had the early symptoms which she confessed to her visiting husband.

We are now, finally, in a position to build up a typical picture of how a heart attack commonly manifests itself. A man who seems to have aged, who has slowed down and become more irritable, may have been pestered by his wife to seek medical attention. He may have begun, for the first time in his life, to have feelings of tightness in the front of his chest and pain in his left shoulder and arm, usually brought on by exercise and relieved by rest.

He has rejected his wife's suggestions, as if the idea of going to the doctor is just what might be expected of a woman. 'You're just a worrier', he will maintain, thus making her into the neurotic member of the partnership and holding onto the picture of himself as someone who never needs doctors.

Then there comes a point when his symptoms change in nature and intensity; he admits to some pain, he may become short of breath, sweating and restless. To begin with, the symptoms can be explained away as severe indigestion. But, as they persist, 'You must let me call the doctor,' his wife eventually entreats.

He may still object: 'I'm not having any doctor near me.'

What happens next, as his condition continues to deteriorate, depends partly on the intensity of the pain, partly on the quality of the marital relationship, partly on the woman's determination and self-assurance, and partly on the presence of others who will support her view.

She calls upon others to see how ill he is. 'Jane and Mrs Brown and I all say you must have a doctor,' she tells him. In the opinion of several people this man is behaving quite irresponsibly, he is carrying his dislike of the medical profession to absurd lengths.

At this point the victim usually capitulates. But there are a few who resist being labelled 'sick' to the very last moment. They won't have an ambulance, insist on going by bus or taxi. Or they keep protesting, 'I'm an impostor', or 'It was only the fish...' If the doctor mentions the diagnosis they will beg, 'Don't say that, Doctor, don't say that.'

Afterwards a wife may draw some comfort and satisfaction from the fact that she had been constantly urging medical care. Thus she can avoid a sense of guilt over having neglected what events have shown was a potentially dangerous condition.

Even severe pain is not an automatic trigger to calling for help or to consenting that help should be called. This sort of pain, in the chest, possibly related to the heart, is so threatening and the accompanying symptoms are so debilitating that a domestic struggle frequently ensues.

We know already, from many studies, that the majority of people treat themselves when they are sick and utilize the advice of others. But, where the developing signs of a heart attack are concerned, the advice itself becomes a serious case for dissension. The process of coming to a decision regarding whether and whence to summon help, what to tell the doctor and at what point he must come, involves a battle of wills in which gains – in terms of the immediate alleviation of pain and distress – have to be balanced against the implications of bidding what could be a last farewell to one's home, one's independence and, possibly, life itself.

3

A modern epidemic

The word 'epidemic' was originally used in relation to devastating outbreaks of infectious disease, caused by some variety of living organism such as viruses or bacteria, and spreading swiftly from one person to another until vast numbers of people were involved. One thinks, for instance, of outbreaks of cholera in the middle of the nineteenth century and of the influenza epidemic or indeed pandemic which spread like wildfire across entire continents after the First World War.

Today, mainly because of improved living standards, we have exchanged the pestilences of the past for diseases which are ultimately just as deadly if less dramatic. Ischaemic heart disease has risen in importance to become the chief cause of death in most countries which enjoy a high standard of living. 'Ischaemia' is a technical term to denote a reduction in blood supply to the heart, the chief manifestations of this disease of modern civilization being heart attacks and angina pectoris.

Until now we have concentrated almost exclusively upon patients' experiences of heart attacks, mediated through the perceptions of those around them.

A MODERN EPIDEMIC

In this chapter we shall be standing back, taking the more detached view of medical scientists who have described what may go wrong with the normal functioning of the heart and the kind of people who seem to be liable to heart attacks.

Our far distant ancestors fell prey to plagues and could even be attacked by wild animals. The contemporary epidemiologist stalks the man-eating tigers of today, which lie in wait for us in our urban jungles or in calm rural retreats. This kind of specialist tries to discover the bodily features and the environments that heart disease patients have in common. Even if the true nature of this deadly cardiac marauder still remains mysterious and elusive, there are tell-tale clues to be found by carefully studying the victims of heart attacks and noting their habitation and their way of life.

So let us first take time to look at that truly extraordinary muscle, the human heart. In the course of an average life-span of seventy-two years over 1,300 million litres of blood will have been pumped around the body by this dynamic organ which is only about the size of a clenched fist. During these years it will have beaten 2,650 million times.

The heart pulsates at a rate of about seventy times a minute, thrusting blood which has been refreshed by oxygen in the lungs throughout the rest of the body and so keeping every part supplied with essential nutrients.

There are four separate chambers in the heart. On both the right and the left sides of a strong dividing wall there are an atrium, or upper entrance hall, and a lower compartment called a ventricle. The right atrium collects all the used, blue blood which has drained back from the body along the veins. It is then passed through a valve into the right ventricle.

This pumping chamber propels the blood off to the lungs, where it loses carbon dioxide and takes up oxygen in exchange. Returning to the left atrium, the oxygenated blood passes on, via another valve, to the left ventricle. The stronger left ventricle forcefully pumps the bright red blood under pressure into the body's main artery, the aorta, whence it is squeezed through all the large and small arteries down to the very smallest vessels, or capillaries. This succession of events within the heart goes to make up one pulsation.

The pace of the heart's beat is regulated by an electrical timing and conducting device which is incorporated centrally in the heart muscle.

At rest the adult heart has to deal with about five litres of blood every minute, but it can increase its output three fold on exercise. It must maintain a constant flow, so as to supply all the body organs with a steady supply of sufficient oxygenated blood to keep them alive, and it must have the capacity to respond rapidly to all kinds of changes in the body's requirements. A certain pressure level is necessary, for instance. The term 'blood pressure' simply refers to the level of pressure in the arterial system and is usually measured by an instrument, a sphygmomanometer, applied around the arm and used by the doctor or nurse in conjunction with a stethoscope.

The heart is not only remarkable as a super-efficient mechanical pump. When scrutinized very closely through an electron-microscope, the heart turns out to be made up of a unique kind of individual muscle cells, which differ in appearance from those in the limbs or any other part of the anatomy. The entire heart consists of a large number of muscle strips intertwined together in a highly complicated manner. The muscle cells have the capacity to keep working, alternately shortening and lengthening, throughout our whole life.

Heart failure, as understood by a doctor, means the inability of the heart to do what is expected of it. A doctor looks for various indications that one or other side of the heart is falling short in its performance. Any serious damage to the heart muscle can mean that it fails to work properly as a pump and so does not send out sufficient blood. Eventually the whole body suffers from the shortage of necessary oxygen and food.

The heart is so essential to our survival that its own blood supply is a matter of prime importance. Like other parts of the body the heart muscle needs a regular supply of fresh, oxygenated blood. But it cannot, as might perhaps be supposed, depend for this purpose on the gushing torrents which bathe its own chambers. The heart is nourished by its own special blood vessels, the coronary arteries, whose ramifications carry red blood under suitable pressure down to the smallest bunches of contracting muscle cells.

Now we begin to see why a heart attack is sometimes colloquially termed 'a coronary', because it is often brought about by a diminished flow of blood to the heart muscle through one of the coronary arteries.

When the heart's motion is carefully studied it turns out to consist of rhythmical electrical activity. This can be recorded by an ECG, or electro-cardiogram, an instrument which is extremely helpful in detecting and diagnosing any serious disturbance in the heart's electrical conducting mechanism. This is especially important in cases of possible heart attack.

The kind of symptoms and signs recorded repeatedly in the last two chapters were all suggestive of heart attacks. The additional features of a weak and irregular pulse and a low blood pressure may be enough to make a doctor decide that his patient has had 'a coronary'. At a later stage the ECG will probably indicate definite damage to the heart muscle or the conducting system. It is also particularly useful for maintaining a constant watch on the motion of the damaged heart after an attack so as to warn the patient's medical attendants of complications which might require swift action.

What happens to bring about a heart attack cannot be properly understood, however, without knowing something about a common condition which affects the arteries of a great many people. This is atheroma or atherosclerosis. The term is derived from the Greek words for porridge and thickness and indeed, to the naked eye, the substance in question does seem both thick and creamy. 'Hardening of the arteries' is a common way of describing this condition in ordinary parlance and it is an apt phrase because, as time goes on, calcium is laid down in these damaged vessels. Early patches of yellowish atheroma can be found in the artery walls of children as young as twelve, and the condition extends as age advances. But the rate of development is variable and it is usually only by middle age or later that there are enough of the plaques or patches of atherosclerosis to interfere with the way our arteries are functioning. As we get older we will all have some degree of atherosclerosis but this certainly does not mean we will all have heart attacks.

The mechanism whereby atherosclerosis is related to heart attacks is not at all clear; some people strongly dispute the association and the following summary is certainly an oversimplification. However, if the inside walls of the coronary arteries become seriously affected by these plaques two results could follow. On the one hand, the inside of the blood vessels will be already narrowed because the patches of atheroma are partly occluding them and they will be less able to dilate when necessary. Secondly the blood flow through the coronary arteries may be slowed down and blood clots may form on top of the plaques. Either way, the vital blood supply to the heart muscle could be impaired, either briefly or for a longer period of time.

Looked at on a worldwide scale there does not seem to be convincing evidence that the general occurrence of atherosclerosis in human blood vessels has been markedly increasing of late. Nevertheless, in certain countries, as we shall presently see, there has undoubtedly been an increase in deaths from ischaemic heart disease, especially among men in the 45 – 54 age group.

Although we are concentrating upon the heart here it is necessary to note in passing that the blood vessels to the brain are as liable to be affected by atherosclerosis as the coronary arteries are. Death rates from stroke, however, which involves interference with the blood supply of the brain, have not changed for many years, over the same period that heart attack mortality has been steadily increasing. So there must be more to this matter than meets the eye. Other factors besides atherosclerosis must be operating in the case of heart attacks. If we could tell what these are perhaps we could start to prevent this disease and the deaths and disability it brings.

A final word on the condition called atherosclerosis. It is much less common in other mammals than in man but many animals can be induced to develop plaques of atheroma in their arteries after being fed some time on modified diets.

Now we are in a position to contemplate what happens in the heart to produce the symptoms of ischaemic heart disease. Essentially it is a matter of a reduced blood supply. Almost invariably atherosclerosis of the coronary arteries is present to some degree – frequently a vital blood vessel is only half the diameter it should be. There may sometimes be a clot completely blocking the artery in question.

In an extreme case the reduction in blood flowing to a key portion of the heart muscle may be virtually complete and may mean that the entire electrical system is dangerously disrupted. Instead of beating regularly and steadily in accordance with the reliable messages from its own pacemaker, in the absence of central control separate small sections of the heart muscle all proceed to contract on their own, in a totally uncoordinated and ineffective manner. Instead of pulsating like a pump the heart is then shaking like a jelly or it may come to a complete stop. Extremely swift treatment can reverse this condition and restore the heart to its proper rhythm.

But a limitation in the blood flow is more likely simply to produce what is known as angina. Angina is experienced as a feeling of tightness and pressure across the front of the chest and beneath the breast bone, characteristically brought on by exercise, like walking up a slope or running for a bus. The discomfort which starts in the chest often radiates, upwards into the throat and jaw, where it may produce a choking sensation or seem like toothache, or down the arms. It is more commonly the left arm which is involved by this 'referred pain'. The feeling in the arm and hand may be one of heaviness and tingling rather than pain. Angina usually passes off in about two minutes and even the most severe attacks rarely last more than ten minutes.

As has been recognized for hundreds of years, anginal attacks are liable to be precipitated by emotional stress and excitement. A susceptible person provoked to violent rage is in danger. But climate can have an effect too, and trying to walk against a cold wind after a large meal may bring on the symptoms. Occasionally angina comes on during the night, but this is most unusual.

Most people with angina can expect to live for many years. They soon learn how to avoid attacks or how to control them when they do occur, by stopping in their tracks and by dissolving, under the tongue, a prescribed drug (a form of nitroglycerine) which soon dilates the blood vessels.

But sometimes the development of angina in an individual who has never before experienced it may signal a subsequent heart attack. And, occasionally, if familiar symptoms of angina become noticeably worse than usual or last longer in a patient who has had them for some time it may be a danger signal.

We can now more or less envisage the physical changes within the heart which bring about what a person experiences as a heart attack. Essentially it represents the effect upon the heart muscle of a serious, sustained shortage of blood. A coronary artery becomes so narrowed, in one of the ways we have described, that it produces what is called an infarct or a myocardial infarction.

This is the medical term for a wedge-shaped piece of damage to the heart muscle. It is somewhat more likely to occur on the front of the heart, affecting the left side which houses the main pumping chamber. As a direct consequence of being deprived of oxygen some bundles of muscle fibres actually die. Immediately small branches of nearby arteries force open lots of tiny connecting links in order to compensate as far as possible for the blockage of a key blood vessel. A kind of emergency circulation, or anastomosis as it is called, takes over. There is a switch to a different circuit, as it were. In the course of time, as the process of healing continues, the heart is left with a scar where the original damage occurred.

So much for the medical meaning of heart attacks. Why is it an epidemic and what can we learn from the overall statistics regarding these disabling and often deadly incidents?

Diseases of the heart and circulation now head the list of killers in the developed world. Not only is vascular disease the major cause of death in rich countries but deaths from ischaemic heart disease, or 'heart attack', have been, until very recently, on the increase in almost all Western countries since the time accurate records were first kept, about fifty years ago.

Heart disease is not always fatal. A fifth of new cases lead to death. But it constitutes a major cause of disability which overshadows the lives of millions. The extent of this condition and its continuing spread, so that it is now starting to be a problem in developing countries, can justify our regarding it as the major epidemic disease of our day.

The realization of its importance for entire societies, as well as its devastating impact on individuals and families, has prompted ambitious and costly research programmes. These are undoubtedly supported in part by people who fear that unless something is soon discovered about heart disease their own sudden demise may at any moment reduce them to a cardiac statistic.

The World Health Organization said ten years ago: 'Coronary heart disease is the leading cause of death in developed countries, striking particularly at men in the prime of life. But there is an unacceptable lack of knowledge about its occurrence in the community and its human, social and economic costs.' Since then a tremendous amount of effort has gone into the intensive study of risk factors. The discussion is all in terms of relative probabilities and considers those aspects of a person's internal or external environment which may make it more or less likely that he will have a heart attack.

In the widest, geographical sense heart disease could lay claim to being a disease of civilization since it mainly affects the population of countries with high standards of hygiene, high living standards and good medical care.

Looking at the world picture, there are several European countries, such as France, Sweden and Italy where the death rate from ischaemic heart disease is considerably lower than in Britain. In 1973 Finland had the highest rate in the world for deaths from this cause among men aged 55-64 (1,009 deaths per 100,000). In startling contrast, the rate for Japanese men a few years later (1976) was only 96 per 100,000. Within the British Isles, in the period 1975-76, Scotland had the unenviable distinction of being second in the world league for deaths in men of this age (929 per 100,000). Northern Ireland was close to Scotland (887), the figures for England and Wales were better (731). New Zealand, at 830 per 100,000 and Australia, at 783 per 100,000, were both somewhat worse than the USA (779).

There is no doubt that these differences between countries are real – it is not simply a matter of differing fashions in diagnosis. The clues must lie in the environments and habits of the people who live in one or another country.

What follows now comes mainly from a Governmental advisory committee on diet and from a Report of the Royal College of Physicians of London. Together they published balanced reviews of all the available information in 1974 and 1976 respectively. Their recommendations regarding prevention will come later. I am bound to say that whilst some doctors feel their advice was not nearly radical enough others object forcefully to its dogmatism. But there is no room for dispute about the actual situation as they found it in the United Kingdom.

According to the most recent statistics, 52 per cent of all deaths in men aged forty-five to fifty-four are due to diseases of the heart and blood vessels. More than three-quarters of these take the form of ischaemic heart disease or heart attacks.

Women during their childbearing years are much less likely to have heart disease than men. Under the age of forty there are six male deaths from this cause to one female death. But, after the menopause, women begin to catch up in this deadly contest until, in the very elderly, the risk of dying from ischaemic heart disease is the same for old women as for old men.

There seems to be no clear difference in risk between people living in towns or the country. But the likelihood of having a heart attack increases as one moves from the south of England towards the west and north, with Scotland and Northern Ireland having the worst experience.

A MODERN EPIDEMIC

The possibility of having a heart attack increases with age. There is a peak among middle-aged men, but it can strike from the mid-thirties onwards.

Most heart attacks (as we too also found) occur at home (54 per cent). The majority of the deaths which ensue from an attack are very rapid indeed, taking place within an hour of onset and, in fact, most of these are practically instantaneous. Two-thirds of the fatal attacks are likely to have happened long before any doctor can get near. In a study carried out in one London borough, half the survivors reached hospital about four hours after the onset of the attack. But it was calculated that, even if the delay had been reduced to an hour, 60 per cent of the victims would already have died by then. There is no escaping the fact that heart attacks are the foremost cause of sudden death in Britain today.

Unlike the infections of former times in which one specific germ had to be present before the illness occurred, the causes of heart disease are extremely complex. All research points to a multifactorial condition, requiring the interaction of many different elements in the total picture. A whole group of factors may be combining to produce the manifestations of ischaemic heart disease and the sudden attacks which are its distinctive and disturbing manifestation.

Several of the presumed risk factors are still being hotly debated. But the most important which have been suggested to date are the proportion of certain fats in the diet, cigarette smoking and high blood pressure.

Let us consider diet first. People in Britain get over 40 per cent of their total energy from the fats in their food. Now the proportion of fat in the average diet of countries where heart attacks are rare is about 30 per cent.

The difference does not look large. Eating habits have changed somewhat over the course of around sixty years; early in the century Britons ate about as much fats as people do now in countries with a lower incidence of ischaemic heart disease. We cannot infer with any confidence, however, that there is a direct, causal relationship between heart attack deaths and the nation's eating habits.

But what about the kind of fats we eat? When various countries' diets are compared in more detail it appears that deaths from ischaemic heart disease possibly relate more closely to the amount of 'hard' or 'saturated' fats which are eaten. The fats described in this way are derived from animals, that is to say from dairy products, like butter, cream and cheese, and from the fat in meat. These fats also include lard and some plant products such as chocolate, coconut and hard cooking fat. They have been postulated as being associated with a high death rate from heart attacks.

'Polyunsaturated fats' is the biochemical term for 'soft' fats and many oils. They are present in corn, sunflower and soya oils and in chicken, fish and nuts, except the coconut.

However, there are exceptions to this general tendency for saturated fats to be associated with heart disease. The Masai and the Somali tribes of East Africa eat a high proportion of saturated, animal fats but do not develop coronary heart disease. They are, however, physically very active.

Recent research has suggested that people who derive a lot of their energy from high fibre diets may be partially protected against ischaemic heart disease. The fibre in question does not come from fruit and vegetables, but is the kind present in breakfast cereals. This new research lead is being closely followed up.

What about the significance of cholesterol? Many people will have heard this word mentioned in connection with the heart. In a study which has been going on for thirty years in Framingham in the USA the level of this substance in the blood of the citizens was measured every year, and the risk of middle-aged men having a heart attack rose according to the concentration of cholesterol. However, the cholesterol in their blood did not bear any relationship to that in their diet.

Cholesterol is a substance which, in Western diets, comes mainly from egg yolks, which do not form a predominant part in those diets. But most if not all the cells in the body can make cholesterol – liver cells are especially good at it. The measurement of the cholesterol in the blood happens to be a convenient way of finding out about other key blood constituents called lipoproteins, which come in various sorts and sizes. When figures for blood cholesterol from different countries are compared there is a strong, positive relationship between the average level of cholesterol for that community as a whole and the occurrence of ischaemic heart disease. Furthermore, the average level of cholesterol in the blood of people in a community closely relates to the proportion of the energy which that community derives from the saturated fats in their diet. The comparison, in the main, is between poor and affluent communities. Blood cholesterol levels are, in general, a reflection of national diets and, when the experience of groups of people are compared, those with the highest levels of blood cholesterol have the highest rates for heart attacks. However, it is not justifiable to jump straight from an association to conclusions about a causal effect.

It is possible to devise diets which are low in cholesterol. Not all our cholesterol comes from eggs – the body makes some of it from saturated fats. So substituting poly-unsaturated fats over a prolonged period should alter the situation. The blood level at any one time is not a very good indication of how much cholesterol there is in the body as a whole because this substance moves between the blood and the tissues in the body according to subtle biochemical changes. But the actual blood cholesterol level is easily measurable and it can be lowered by strict diets in experimental groups of people. This requires determination, dedication and conviction on the part of doctors on the one hand and a highly motivated and compliant population on the other.

Trials of this sort have already been carried out and others are still in progress in a number of centres. The results take several years to assess. Regular measurements must be taken of the levels of blood cholesterol in groups who have had a modified diet and in 'control' groups who have been eating what they like, and then the epidemiologists have to stand by and see how many people in each group succumb to heart disease.

But deliberately lowering the blood cholesterol, either by diet or by a drug, has so far produced disappointing results. It is unfortunately by no means proven that altering the composition of someone's diet or energetically aiming to lower his blood cholesterol will guarantee that he avoids a heart attack.

Indeed a number of respected cardiologists and medical scientists are highly sceptical of the part played by saturated fats in producing atherosclerosis. They see no simple and direct relationship between atheroma and heart attacks; they do not believe that dietary modifications can prevent atherosclerotic heart disease in man; and they warn against the danger of adopting unnatural diets (high in soft margarine, for instance) without calculating their possible side effects. Some of the most recent clinical trials have shown their forebodings to be justified.

If this whole dietary story sounds extremely bewildering and deeply depressing you may take comfort on two counts. Firstly, the prevailing confusion amongst experts simply demonstrates that the full explanation of heart attacks is definitely still eluding us. Secondly, even in people with very high blood cholesterol levels, the actual number who will not develop heart disease in the next ten or twenty years greatly exceeds the number of those who will.

With smoking, the picture is somewhat clearer. More than half the excess mortality that smokers experience as compared to non-smokers comes in the form of cardiovascular disease. Looked at another way, about a quarter of the 40,000 yearly deaths in men and women under sixty-five from heart disease are closely associated with cigarette smoking. Ten thousand cardiac deaths a year are partly attributed, therefore, to smoking. Or the risk for smokers of dying from ischaemic heart disease is twice that of non-smokers. It is unusual for a non-smoker under the age of forty-five to die from ischaemic heart disease.

On the whole, however, smoking has an even worse effect on people whose arterial disease affects other blood vessels – in the aorta, the body's main artery, or in the fingers and toes. But smoking twenty cigarettes a day does double the risk of having a heart attack.

People whose blood pressure is above the optimal level for their age and sex are more likely to have a heart attack. I shall not detail the levels of blood pressure in question – for one thing, there are differences in measurements according to the circumstances in which they are made. The risk of heart disease steadily increases with increasing blood pressure. But the effect is much greater if the person is a smoker or has a raised blood cholesterol level.

Risks multiply when they occur together. It seems as if it is not a matter of simple addition of the risk factors. Taken together, therefore, a rough and ready measure can be made of how susceptible a population or a person is to heart disease. But this kind of prediction, in the case of a particular individual, still remains very imprecise. No doctor can say with certainty to one patient, 'You will have a heart attack' and to another, 'You will not.'

Obesity is a difficult topic. When *is* someone 'obese', for instance? Its relationship with heart disease is closely tied up with the varied dietary factors already dealt with. There is evidence that substantial weight reduction alone will reduce the higher death rate from many of the different conditions, including heart attack, which fat people risk.

Within the United Kingdom as a whole, the death rate from heart disease is highest where the local water supply is soft and lowest in places using hard water.

Diabetics in Western cultures are more liable to have heart attacks than non-diabetics, the difference being most striking for women patients. But this does not apply in the case of Japanese or Africans. Anti-diabetic treatment, in its present form at least, does not seem to reduce the diabetic patient's greater risk of ischaemic heart disease.

Accounts of the effect of alcohol on ischaemic heart disease were contradictory at first. In moderate quantities, it appears to have a protective effect, although prolonged, excessive intake of alcohol can produce a recognizable form of heart failure.

There is general agreement that people in Britain have become increasingly sedentary. However, in a part of Finland with the highest death rate from heart attacks in the world, heavy physical work does not seem to protect men who are already at risk for other reasons. Postmen in Britain have far fewer heart attacks than postal clerks.

Exercise must be vigorous in order to be protective, improving the level of performance of both the heart and the lungs. The research which showed a relationship between cereals and heart attacks indicated that a high fibre dietary energy intake was associated with a lowered risk of heart attacks. Since energy intake increases with physical activity the importance of both exercise and fibre in the diet cannot be ignored.

It is estimated that the contraceptive pill increases the risk of a heart attack by three times in women over forty. It will be recalled that women are presently in a much safer situation than men, at least until after the menopause. But heavy cigarette smokers (over twenty a day) who are also on the pill are seriously increasing their risk of heart disease.

Certain families run an abnormally high risk of heart attacks because of a rare congenital condition. This manifests itself in early childhood as an abnormally high level of cholesterol in the blood.

The role of stress in provoking heart attacks has been reported from America and some other countries. The people concerned are said to manifest what is called 'Type A' behaviour. They are ambitious, aggressive and assertive, preoccupied with deadlines and anxious to achieve a great deal in a short time.

This is a difficult idea to test experimentally, for all kinds of reasons. But even if it may not be possible to demonstrate that frustration and anxiety bring about the mysterious condition which doctors call ischaemic heart disease, it is not difficult to imagine that emotion might play a part in precipitating at least some attacks. In this connection it is perhaps worth mentioning that those recently widowed have been shown to have a higher than average risk of themselves falling victims to heart attacks. So death from 'a broken heart' may occasionally be a reality.

Perhaps I can end this chapter on a more cheerful note. It was lately observed in America that, over the period 1968-76, death rates from all causes had begun to show a decline. But the change in the death rates from heart attacks was the most dramatic feature, affecting both men and women and most age groups. However, the attacks themselves have not declined in frequency. So there is the same amount of illness from ischaemic heart disease but fewer deaths from it.

The reasons for this welcome state of affairs are uncertain. It may be that health-conscious Americans have already modified their life styles sufficiently to change their life chances. This is strongly argued by American epidemiologists, who maintain that it is only necessary to reduce each of a whole series of risks by a small amount to improve the overall picture significantly. However, the drop in death rates could already be detected by 1963, years before the enthusiasm for jogging and dieting had begun.

There are very early signs of something similar in the way of lower death rates from heart disease in other countries too. Time alone will show whether and why the great epidemic is on the wane.

4

Treatment options

Earlier in this book I gave examples of how people had tried to deal with a heart attack on their own. Some of their problems arose from puzzlement regarding the symptoms with which they were confronted. But they were also unsure what to do in the way of first aid. Finally, they had to decide what was the most appropriate kind of outside, expert help and how to get that help quickly.

Anyone wishing to acquire the skills of cardiac resuscitation must learn them in a setting which allows supervision and practical training – such as via the Red Cross.

Some cardiologists are convinced that many more people should know how to cope if someone collapses with a heart attack. In certain American cities a massive drive has already begun to provide many groups in the population with the basic skills to keep a heart attack victim's brain supplied with oxygen even if his heart appears to have stopped. The best-known experiment of this kind is in Seattle where responsibility for dealing with cardiac emergencies lies with the fire services who are providing instruction for citizens interested in this kind of first aid. At present the only place in

TREATMENT OPTIONS

Britain where this kind of training is being positively canvassed is Brighton, where the Cardiac Ambulance Service has taken on the job of running classes in places of work.

But there are certain key things to look out for which will help you decide whether you may actually be experiencing or witnessing a heart attack and what you should do whilst waiting for medical assistance.

In this connection it is worth thinking of the American term, 'the executive wife', which draws attention to the fact that it is very often women who have to deal with these events. The woman who is present must be prepared to take firm control of the situation and trust her own judgement, remembering always that it is better to be safe than sorry.

If you make a mistake and call the doctor or the ambulance for someone who, on careful medical examination, turns out not to be having a heart attack no harm has been done. You cannot be expected to be an expert in cardiac diagnosis. So do not be afraid to err on the safe side when delay could cost someone's life.

Let us first dispose of some common sensations and symptoms which are almost certainly not signs of a heart attack. The first of these is what is known as 'palpitations'.

This is a sense of awareness of the heart's motion. It may seem to be pounding hard or its rate may seem to have changed. Such a sensation is perfectly natural if you have a fright or sudden excitement. It has passed into everyday speech in such telling expressions as 'My heart missed a beat' or 'His heart leapt at the news'.

But awareness of the heart's motion may also come about without any obvious external cause for alarm or joy. If you simply begin to think about it you can often start noticing your own heartbeats. Worrying about your heart is liable to make you especially conscious of its movements. And anxiety or nervous strain of any kind may cause someone to have 'palpitations'.

Some kind of variation in the rate of the heartbeat or pulse is perfectly normal. It is related to breathing, for instance, speeding up as you breathe in. Then the heart rate has to increase with exercise, to ensure that sufficient blood will get to the muscles and supply the additional energy they require. We saw how the heart was uniquely fitted to act as a pump which would reliably respond to changes in the body's requirements.

So, although the heart's rate at rest is about seventy beats per minute, either sudden fright or exercise will naturally increase it. You should also remember that children have faster heart rates than adults. But we can fortunately leave them out of the heart attack picture.

It is also quite common to experience what doctors call 'occasional extrasystoles', the feeling of an extra beat with a longer pause after it. There may even be a succession of these odd beats over the course of a short period of time. Again, if you are concentrating upon your heart, you are more likely to be aware of them.

While you may have become anxious about your heart rhythm or rate and may wish to tell your doctor about it so that he or she can build this information into an assessment of your general health, none of the symptoms we have mentioned are, by themselves, a reason for summoning a doctor to the spot. Mere awareness of the beating of the heart is not a sign of heart attack.

What about pains in the chest? Here we are on more difficult ground because there are all kinds of reasons, short of a heart attack or angina, why someone should have a pain in the chest. It could come from the ribs, or the muscles, or from the nerves in the skin of the chest wall. It could originate in the covering of the lungs or in the gullet. There are, furthermore, different kinds of pain in the chest.

Pain is notoriously difficult to communicate to another person. Its nature is intensely personal. All the same, most people can roughly sort out certain varieties of pain. A short, sharp, stabbing pain in the left side of the chest is quite commonly complained of by healthy young people. It comes on arbitrarily, without any connection with exercise or eating or deep breathing and it is of no significance whatsoever. This kind of chest pain is not a sign of underlying heart disease.

The young may have a sore chest after violent contact sports. In these cases the precise position of the pain can usually be located and is simply due to minor bruising. Of course, the pain of a broken rib is a different matter, but circumstances should clarify this possibility.

It should be clear from the last chapter that a heart attack is mainly a condition of middle age and over. Now there are disagreements about when 'middle' age begins, and the older we are ourselves the later it starts and the longer it seems to last. But, for practical purposes, you can assume that heart pain does not arise before the mid-thirties. In fact women, who live on average longer than men and have, as we saw, a different experience where heart disease is concerned, are unlikely to have cardiac pain before their forties.

The first-hand accounts of patients earlier in this book showed how they described their chest pain. Some of them had already been under treatment for angina. Others were clearly experiencing angina for the first time in the period which later events proved was preceding a heart attack.

If someone experiences a sensation of tightness and oppression in the front of the chest brought on by exercise, usually walking and especially up a slope or upstairs, it could be from the heart. This sort of pain, possibly spreading up into the face and neck or down the left arm, does not last long. It is over in a few minutes. Stopping whatever one is doing and resting generally stops the pain. It is not a persistent pain though it may be a recurrent one.

If you or a person whom you know begins to suffer from this kind of pain for the first time a doctor should be told about it. He or she will make the necessary investigations and prescribe treatment. The doctor should be able to decide whether or not the symptoms are due to angina, that is to say a temporary reduction in blood to the heart muscle, or if they are of more serious import. If you are in any doubt, tell your doctor early rather than late about this kind of pain.

Now we come to the symptoms suggestive of a heart attack.

The pain of a heart attack is characteristically felt as a sensation of great pressure in the chest. There is a feeling of squeezing, as though a band was being tightened round the ribs. These unpleasant and painful sensations are centred beneath the breastbone. They are persistent and severe. Although they may ease somewhat, they return and become worse and worse until they reach a kind of plateau.

As may happen with angina, there is often a feeling of heaviness and painful aching in the shoulders and arms, more commonly affecting the left side. These symptoms may spread right down to the hand. Or the pain may extend upwards into the throat, neck and jaw.

Pain is rarely the only feature. Usually there is also

TREATMENT OPTIONS

shortness of breath, although the person has no reason to be breathless because he is not, as a rule, exerting himself at the time. The breathing is shallow and rapid, but there is no cough.

The stomach can be affected too, causing nausea and vomiting. As we have seen, people are frequently inclined to think first in terms of a particularly severe bout of indigestion.

The victim may perspire profusely, until his clothes are drenched in sweat.

The change in facial colour and general appearance is often striking. A patient can look pale or greyish.

Dizziness, not in itself a cardiac symptom, is something to look out for when combined with sudden chest pain. The person may simply feel light-headed. Or he may slump to the ground and seem to be losing consciousness.

The person having a heart attack may feel intensely apprehensive, however much he may try to conceal it from others.

If you are present when someone is showing these signs of illness try to persuade him to lie flat. Do not, on any account, encourage or force him to take exercise, for example like climbing stairs.

If the heart is in difficulty the brain can become dangerously short of oxygen and it can be helped if the person's head is low. Do not try to prop him up. It is better that he should lie or sprawl upon the ground than be shoved into a semblance of sitting.

Forget about changing his clothes and cleaning him up. That can come later. Do not bother about a doctor seeing someone in a dirty or dishevelled state – the doctor can take it.

Feel for the patient's pulse, at the wrist or to one side of the throat. If it is difficult to detect or seems irregular this is a further reason for very rapid action.

By now you should have enough clues to impress you with the seriousness of the situation. Phone for the ambulance at once. Do not hesitate to use a neighbour's phone or one in a shop or work place.

If you have the help of one other person, get him or her to stay with the patient while you make absolutely sure that your 999 emergency call is understood. Then change places and have your 'assistant' wait outside the building so that the ambulance men will know exactly where to come and will waste no time when they arrive.

The advice I have given above is for the most serious case, when someone has collapsed. An ambulance will bring medical aid fast. In some places, as we shall see presently, there are cardiac ambulances. But, once you have made up your mind that you think someone is collapsing from a heart attack, the important thing is to get this message clearly to the source of rapid aid. If there is a special cardiac ambulance in your area it will be sent if the message seems to justify it.

Of course, as we saw in the early chapters, the symptoms may be considerably more uncertain and confusing. Then you would do best to phone your own doctor.

When you get through to whoever answers, it is once again very important indeed that you should give a clear, concise account of what you have noticed. If the patient has mentioned the sort of persistent pressing chest pain we have described, be sure that you mention it. You must also be certain to describe any shortness of breath, sweating and dizziness, if these are present.

Do not fail to convey a sense of urgency if you yourself

feel it. Remember that the person receiving your call has not seen what you have seen and does not know what you know. Only you can paint a vivid word picture of what is happening on the scene. This can be just as truly an emergency as any accident. Get the message through clearly. If you are really worried, say so and say why.

Doctors and their receptionists are alert to the possibility that patients and relatives may interpret a heart attack as severe indigestion. But, if you know that there are other symptoms present of the kind described as well as what seem like stomach troubles, do not fail to pass on these other tell-tale signs.

Of course doctors and ambulance men do not want to be called out unnecessarily. But relatives and members of the public should not hesitate to call for medical assistance when a person of middle age or over suddenly takes ill with the kind of complaints and signs we have listed.

The indications for summoning immediate help should be especially clear for people who are known to have ischaemic heart disease, manifested by angina for instance, and those who have already had one heart attack. Relatives of such people must carry the uncomfortable knowledge that one day or night they may have to deal with an episode like this. If you feel sufficiently strongly about it you may wish to prepare yourself in a more positive fashion, by taking instruction in cardiac resuscitation.

But there is a danger here which must be mentioned. At the present time in England, out of every 1,000 thirty-year-old men, seventy-five will die of ischaemic heart disease before retirement age. About forty-five of these deaths will take place without any medically trained person being present. Even intensive coronary care may only be able to save a few lives out of the seventy-five.

So supposing you do everything humanly possible – you take training in life-saving techniques, you are spot-on with the diagnosis and you send for expert help quickly – but it is all in vain. Supposing the person dies before your eyes, who will you blame? If the victim is your husband or your father or someone else close to you, you are certain to go through a stage of reliving and questioning your own and other people's behaviour at the time of the disaster. It is very likely that, as part of this process, you will come to blame yourself for what you did or did not do at the time.

Try to remember that you may be face to face with fate. Quite possibly no one, at that time, could have made a difference to the outcome; the attack was simply too sudden or too severe.

But we are concerned in this book with the survivors of heart attacks. Seventy per cent of those suffering a heart attack will be alive one month later and, as has been stressed, the danger of death is highest shortly after the attack, in the first twenty-four hours. After forty-eight hours the risk rapidly declines.

What kinds of treatment are likely to be offered to someone who has called for medical help?

The answer depends, firstly, on where the patient resides. There are a number of treatment options open but they are not uniform throughout any country and there is not yet full agreement amongst doctors and cardiologists about the optimal place of treatment. The main division is between home and hospital treatment. But, in hospital, patients may or may not enter an intensive coronary care unit. They may be cared for in a normal ward. And, in some places, special emergency resuscitation measures may be applied to patients in the ambulance going to hospital, or as soon as they reach the accident and emergency department.

Put this way it might sound as though someone's chances are arbitrary and unfairly determined by where they live. Some people may feel indignant because coronary care units are not widely available; they may wonder why cardiac ambulances are not the rule rather than the exception, and they may be very surprised to learn of heart attacks ever being treated at home.

But it is only in the past fifteen years that intensive coronary care units have been established. Before then people were all treated at home or in a general ward. Surprisingly, we are still not certain exactly how much these units have contributed to the saving of lives. Perhaps they have reduced the death rate from ischaemic heart disease in men before retirement age by about 5 per cent. Put in terms of numbers, intensive coronary care may save the lives of three or four out of every thousand middle-aged men.

Since coronary care units were introduced in some hospitals, admission rates in general for heart attacks have gone up and up. But the numbers of deaths of people in hospital from ischaemic heart disease have remained about the same. There is some evidence that more of the milder cases are being admitted to hospital now. In addition deaths are being partly kept down by the superior treatments now available in hospital.

Coronary care units were set up with the aim of treating people whose hearts were fibrillating as a result of an attack. This totally uncoordinated and inefficient contracting of the heart can be reversed by the swift application of an electric current. The central idea of such a coronary unit is that patients there can be constantly monitored. At the first sign of a cardiac arrest the staff can rush in and restart the heart which has stopped. All the equipment is conveniently to hand, the staff are all specially trained and there is an unusually high ratio of nurses to patients.

Other special forms of treatment are also administered, for controlling pain and for improving and sustaining the function of the heart in a number of ways.

Apart from the monitoring and treatment facilities associated with a coronary care unit, precise diagnosis of the stage and extent of the ischaemic heart disease can be made. This is done both from the evidence provided by the electrocardiogram to which the patients are connected and from biochemical investigation of their blood for certain chemical enzymes which are produced when the heart muscle suffers serious damage. A great deal of basic research into cardiac disease has been made possible by the existence of these extremely costly treatment units. But the main justification for them is that they ensure rapid resuscitation.

Just as the relatives and other witnesses to a heart attack have to think first in terms of the aid they themselves can offer and then in terms of obtaining medical aid, so doctors and those watching over the provision of medical aid must decide what is most appropriate.

Wherever patients are cared for there should be the means to hand to deal with the heart rhythm failing. A doctor who rushes to a patient's side because of an emergency call can do a lot to calm the victim and to ease his or her pain. But, without special equipment, the doctor himself can only perform first aid in the way of resuscitation. Granted that the doctor will be more skilled in this procedure than the lay person, this action, if it becomes necessary, can still only gain a little more time.

Supposing an ambulance turns up, all ready to rush a patient to hospital. If the patient's heart is arrested by the time the ambulance turns up or if it stops in the ambulance, without special defibrillating equipment the ambulance crew will be facing the same dilemma. They only have their bare hands.

It is for these reasons that some cardiologists, in different parts of the British Isles and elsewhere, have been thinking in terms of providing special ambulances whose crews have sufficient knowledge and means to perform cardiac resuscitation on the spot, whenever someone is struck down. A further, logical development of the same ideas would lead to more GPs having the equipment and the motivation to take care of heart attack patients in their own homes.

The value of cardiac ambulances is strictly limited by geography. Unless they can get rapidly to a heart attack victim who is liable to develop fibrillation or who has developed it, there is no point in having them. If there is delay in navigating busy traffic or if the victim is more than a certain distance from the base where the ambulance is kept, this expensive special facility is quite worthless.

In Brighton, England, the cardiac ambulances can be directly summoned by a member of the public, by dialling 999. They are manned not by doctors but by ambulance men who have had an intensive theoretical and practical course in cardiac resuscitation using a portable defibrillator. Meanwhile, as mentioned before, ordinary people in Brighton are being encouraged to take classes in cardiac first aid, arranged in factories and offices, so that they can keep a heart artificially pumping until it either recovers on its own or until the ambulance men can galvanize it into action.

In Belfast, Northern Ireland, another city whose modest size makes the ambulance trip between home and hospital relatively short, a special mobile coronary care unit is in operation. The crew in this case does not consist of paramedicals. Instead a junior doctor (or medical student) and a nurse are available to take the necessary apparatus directly to the patient's home, as soon as a call from a doctor or a member of the public is received. Half the patients are reached within ten minutes and, after emergency treatment, they are transferred to the coronary care unit of the hospital.

A study carried out in Bristol, England, in the early 1970s first cast doubt on the superiority of intensive coronary care over home care. Until then it had been taken for granted that the outcome of hospital-based treatment was necessarily better and that it was virtually negligent not to provide it. But the 1976 investigation showed that, when patients were more or less randomly allocated to home or hospital care, the outcome in terms of deaths after twenty-eight days did not seem to be strikingly different. Not only is there still hot debate about this topic but it is not at all easy to resolve the issue.

We have seen how, when a heart attack is sudden and the symptoms are intense, most people send for help well within an hour. But, if it is a GP who is told, he or she may be bound to take another half an hour to reach the patient. Then there can be fifteen minutes to half an hour whilst the doctor makes a diagnosis and begins the treatment. If the doctor decides to call an ambulance, more time elapses before it arrives. Finally comes the journey to hospital. The whole process, from onset to admission, may take around three hours. So the person who gets to hospital may have

TREATMENT OPTIONS

already passed the most dangerous point and be fairly likely to survive.

We must add to these time-tabling considerations the fact that it is the responsibility of the individual GP to make up his or her mind about whether to treat a particular case at home or transfer the patient to hospital. It is not possible for any investigator to dictate to doctors how they will manage their cases. So a completely random allocation cannot be arranged.

Nevertheless, cardiologists in Teesside, in the north-east of England, carefully monitored the way in which all suspected heart attacks were dealt with during one year. They managed to secure total cooperation from all the doctors and hospitals and from every trained person who might encounter an attack. Then virtually every patient was interviewed.

In the course of very detailed analysis, which is too complex to summarize here, they separated home-treated cases from those which were sent to a coronary care unit or to an ordinary hospital ward. In terms of severity the cases were all very similar. Some doctors were in the habit of sending all their cases into hospital, others had a mixed policy. Not surprisingly the fatality amongst patients was related to the severity of their attack. The death rates among those treated at home were lower than those treated in hospital.

The Teesside cardiologists finally recommended that patients might be left at home if there had been a delay of two or three hours before the general practitioner arrived. In fact, for people who survived to come into care, they thought home care was as good as if not better than hospital treatment. But they were absolutely emphatic that, wherever patients were cared for, there should be equipment available to deal with cardiac arrest as well as appropriate pain killers and tranquillizers. Doctors on Teesside are now being positively encouraged to arrange matters so that they have easy access to all the necessary drugs and electrical equipment. They are being encouraged to stay with those heart attack patients whom they may decide to treat at home, watching them carefully, if necessary for a number of hours, until the acute danger period is past.

Unfortunately therefore, even the matter of immediate treatment for heart attacks has not been finally resolved. The deaths which occur amongst those who are admitted to a coronary care unit largely depend on the age of the patients, their general health and the stage after the attack at which they come into care.

From the patients' point of view there is no certainty about what the form and place of treatment will be, even when medical aid does appear on the scene. The pattern is changing, as cardiologists and doctors modify their attitudes and as the idea of community care becomes acceptable to more people.

For a time it looked as if coronary care units were 'the answer'. Now that much more research has been done and different experiments in the delivery of cardiac care are being evaluated there is a strong move towards making emergency treatments available on the spot. This will involve the primary care doctor even more than at present and will require many women to extend their role as the patients' primary source of succour and comfort. Some futurologists even envisage a time when it might be feasible for patients or their attendants to administer electrical first aid to the heart themselves.

But, in the meantime, the best that patients and their relatives and helpers can do is to sound the alarm loud and clear whenever they suspect an attack. Then they must trust themselves to the medical services in their area.

5

Recovery

Contrary to popular belief the human heart is very strong indeed and has great powers of recovery after an attack. The process of healing in the damaged muscle begins soon after the acute episode. First, special white blood cells appear on the scene and remove the dead muscle fibres. About twelve days later elastic-like collagen fibres are already being laid down in the affected area. As these fibres knit together they form a firm scar. The whole process is completed in two months.

Meanwhile, the patient's general physical condition improves markedly after the first forty-eight hours when the risk of complications is largely over. Doctors now encourage people to get up early, often after a mere two days in bed.

The regimes used today are in marked contrast to those which prevailed for many years prior to the 1950s. Previously doctors used to recommend prolonged bed rest, on the theory that the heart was rather like a broken bone and needed immobilizing. It is of course impossible to rest the heart without stopping it completely. Fortunately for us it persists in beating steadily and sustaining every other part of the body. Resting a patient for a prolonged period of time actually had the direst consequences, reducing a formerly active, confident individual to miserable, passive invalidism. Their long-term recovery was very seriously imperilled by such undue caution. Lying in bed with nothing to do but contemplate the sorry state to which they had been reduced, patients became deeply depressed and dubious of their ability ever to return to a semblance of normal living.

Doctors nowadays know that getting someone moving soon does not carry any risk. The heart will not burst or develop leaks or bulges. An uncomplicated case can be treated at home, provided good nursing care, by family and health professionals, is available.

It is reckoned that perhaps as many as half the infarcts which occur in people's hearts happen without the symptoms ever being recognized as those of a heart attack. In such silent or missed cases, when neither the patients nor their doctors have realized what was happening, there may well have been no rest in bed whatsoever. Yet, years later perhaps, signs of an old scar may be incidentally found in the course of a medical examination.

But old medical ideas die hard. Indeed they often persist in the popular imagination long after they have been discarded by doctors. So people may carry notions about treatments for heart attacks which they picked up from their parents' generation and may then return to old, remembered rituals as a reassuring way of coping with new crises.

When I was a medical undergraduate a famous Edinburgh cardiologist used to pounce ferociously upon any student who dared to mutter something about a patient possibly having a weak heart.

'The diagnosis of a weak heart,' he would thunder, 'is a weak diagnosis. Talk of a tired heart is the talk of a tired doctor.' Whilst he may have succeeded in impressing strict habits of cardiac examination and nomenclature upon us as future doctors, potential patients who lacked the benefit of his tutelage would be liable to go on thinking in outmoded terms.

Nowadays patients may be discharged from hospital in ten days. If they have been initially admitted to a coronary care unit, they are usually moved out of this intensely supervised setting into a neighbouring general ward in two days for the start of their convalescence. A new generation of young hospital visitors is growing up who will probably no longer associate heart attacks with the picture of someone spending weeks and weeks in bed, 'taking it easy'.

Although the immediate treatment of heart attacks has changed to a 'get up and go' approach the entire experience still leaves relatives and patients bewildered. Time and again, accounts of how patients have fared after an attack repeat the themes of denial, depression and confused uncertainty. It seems as if doctors, with the best will in the world and with far more confidence in the heart's recuperative powers than their predecessors, are still often out of touch with the day-to-day concerns which preoccupy their patients throughout the weeks and months immediately following an attack. It has taken many separate studies of the successes and pitfalls of rehabilitation to bring medical attention to bear on this very important topic.

The process of recovery, physical, emotional and social, is an extended open-ended affair, lacking the drama of early life-saving procedures or the intellectual fascination which physicians derive from differential diagnosis. Until recently the great bulk of cardiac research has been directed towards detailed biochemical aspects of the heart's functioning in health and disease, with the entirely laudable aim of unravelling the causes of this contemporary epidemic. Much less attention and time has been given to finding out how ordinary patients and their families come to terms with a life-threatening event of this magnitude and cope with its reverberations.

However, a great deal of work has now been done in New England and in Britain, following up patients at intervals after a heart attack, to find out how they have rearranged their lives and their changed circumstances. Are there any gaps which need attention in the services provided to aid the rehabilitation of heart attack patients?

It may sound as though all the patients were men, but this is simply because practically all the studies so far carried out have in fact concentrated on male heart attack cases and their wives.

The survivor of a heart attack can expect to experience powerful and disturbing emotions. At the beginning, his pain and weakness are not only frightening in themselves but carry the threat of imminent death. As the people around him display undisguised alarm and concern and as medical help is hastily enlisted the person in the centre of the drama feels his own deepest fears confirmed by their behaviour. The urgency of their actions reflects the anxiety he is trying to repress whilst at the same time he desperately needs some ease for his immediate physical symptoms. The dulling of pain which is achieved by the administration of morphine and tranquillizers usually brings an immense feeling of relief and allows someone who may have struggled hard against the gathering forces of his attack to subside at last into the comforting passivity of patienthood.

The first few hours of intense or intensive care, wherever

they take place, are likely to pass in a rush of emergency treatments and tests. A journey from home is involved for many who are thus obliged to relinquish the comforting familiarity of their own beds for attachment to the latest manifestations of high medical technology.

Some patients who enter coronary care units find them alarming places. They may feel both isolated and under continual scrutiny. Patients are often nursed in separate, glass-walled cubicles through whose transparent fronts they can not only be seen by the staff but can also glimpse the nurses hastening to attend to the needs of other people whose condition may be even more parlous than their own.

But many patients find the first forty-eight hours a time for reflecting on their own remarkable good fortune. They are the lucky ones, the survivors, snatched from death. The appliances with which they are surrounded and monitored convey a welcome sense of security. Frequently they declare, 'This is the best possible place to be' and they may well imagine that the electro-cardiogram leads by which they are connected to the monitoring machine are actually conveying a positive health-giving current in their direction. The armamentarium of a cardiology unit is a source of reassurance, proof of the power of modern medicine to save lives and heal men's hearts. The hospital bed is a warm cocoon from within which they can receive the merited congratulations and commiserations of relatives and friends.

Even at this stage, however, some niggling doubts and worries may begin to intrude. The fact that their families are clearly managing without them is disturbing as well as comforting since it demonstrates that they themselves were not indispensable after all. And the sense of being lucky to be alive can provide only modified and transient euphoria mixed as it is with medical evidence that something did after all go seriously wrong with their own heart.

We get so used to medical terms like 'anxiety' and 'depression' for describing people's states of mind that we forget the original meaning of some familiar words. 'Fainthearted' sums up very well the special fears and hesitancies which follow a heart attack. It is not surprising that those who have experienced such an assault should feel 'brokenhearted'. Many patients are both sad and fearful, grieving and worried.

An event like this brings home to people the unwelcome realization of their own mortality. Being so very close to death, even though they have escaped, is a most disturbing experience. The possibility of another attack is difficult to forget. Nevertheless, about a quarter of the people having a first heart attack deny that they experienced any particular apprehension from the time of onset of their symptoms right throughout their stay in hospital. These patients manage to avoid any anxiety or depression and they return rapidly to work. It is clearly a tremendous advantage to be able to minimize the significance of an attack and to go on pretty much as before.

But it is commoner for a patient to experience at least some worry over what life will be like after an attack and to regret the passing of the years of confident health and vigour. They wonder whether they will ever be the same again, whether they will be able to hold down their jobs and satisfy their wives and manage the household as before.

They want to know exactly what has happened to their heart to reduce them suddenly to such a humiliating posture of dependence on others. How long will this demoralizing situation last? What exactly will they be able to do when they get home? Should they be specially cautious? Even though nowadays the hospital stay is not long in real terms it is sufficient to allow time for sombre reflection. Behind many such apparently straightforward requests for factual information is the more fundamental question, 'Why did this happen to me?' People search for some explanation for their own singular misfortune, in order to render it both more acceptable and more manageable. If they are not merely pawns of inscrutable or arbitrary fate, if they can discover some reason for their own personal attack, they may be able to take evasive action in future.

It is all very well to feel initially that one has been lucky. But reason forces the realization that luck could just as easily turn the other way. It is obviously desirable to discover what seems to have been the cause of this attack so that the provoking circumstances can be modified or avoided in the future. In our culture at least, people feel a very strong urge to believe that they, or their doctors, can control their fate. So they beg earnestly for advice on the future management of their lives, wishing for reassuring rituals and regimens whose observance can lessen their fears.

Confined in hospital, with time on their hands for perhaps the first occasion in years, patients try to fit what has just befallen them into a meaningful picture of their whole lives. This desire for understanding is a feature of every serious illness. When someone's heart has been attacked it can inflict a serious blow to their former sense of themselves as someone invulnerable, never ill, always able to cope. It demands an explanation phrased in terms of something unwise which they did or some precaution they did not take. The advice they want now must be couched in terms of avoiding future ills.

The heart is central to our whole physical and psychological self-image. It is not only known to control our bodies but it is bound up with ideas of our strength and our most powerful emotions. So damage to the heart may well seem to strike at the core of personality and achievement both in the fields of work and in areas of life where feelings and attachments predominate. Men generally do not want to be seen as soft-hearted or weak-hearted. To visualize any kind of damage to the heart can be dreadfully threatening, challenging one's self-conception and raising doubts about future performance in a whole range of roles.

As I have said, doctors take a very positive, optimistic stance with regard to mobilization after a heart attack and aim to give patients the minimum time to lie around contemplating what they wrongly imagine may be a much restricted future. There is no good medical reason for keeping patients who have had no complications in bed for longer than two days. Thereafter they can gradually resume normal activities, with the ultimate aim of returning to work and normal functioning.

Indeed the patient himself may feel relatively confident at the point of discharge. Having made steady progress and moved, possibly, from initial intensive care to management in an ordinary ward, he has received physiotherapy and been encouraged in undertaking regular, graded activities. He will have been surrounded by nurses and doctors who take complete recovery for granted. Some hospitals issue guidance leaflets to patients who have had a heart attack, listing the ways in which they can modify their habits with the aim of improving their general health and lessening the chances of further cardiac trouble.

But, once patients get back home – or, if they have been

nursed at home, once the first stage of close medical supervision is past – they are in a very different situation. Now, instead of being surrounded by doctors and nurses who 'know' what the patients should or should not do, they are back with their families who are considerably less confident. It is here that many difficulties have to be faced, often without sufficient support either from professionals or from others who are similarly placed.

In the first two chapters we saw some of the conflicts arising at the very moment that an attack was engulfing a reluctant patient, how some men were desperately struggling against the relinquishment of their normal roles and familiar patterns of behaviour. At that point it must have seemed that matters could go either way. The trouble could turn out to be trivial, in which case all the fuss their wives were making would be shown to be unnecessary.

But, by the time the heart patient is back in circulation he enters a totally different domestic scene. Those who were alarmed and who had urged the need for help have been abundantly proved right. Events have demonstrated man's frailty. The fragility of human hopes and the ever-present danger of death, which most of us sensibly and conveniently ignore most of the time, have been dramatically and literally brought home to the entire family.

Throughout our lives our own view of ourselves is inextricably bound up with the opinion others hold. It is in face-to-face encounters that we are recognized and feel ourselves to be distinct and valuable persons. Our own identity is partly formed as well as reflected in the picture others form of us. We cannot understand people fully apart from their social context or setting. So the conception a heart patient has of himself will be closely bound up with the ideas which his wife and his friends and his employer hold about his capabilities.

Clearly, therefore, it would help if everyone was just as positive and optimistic as the most up-to-date physicians. But, inevitably, lay notions of what can be expected of someone recovering from a heart attack are liable to differ from professional judgements.

The difficulty is further compounded by the fact that the wife and family have so recently been proved right in their cautious assessment of the patient's health. After what may have been weeks or more of trying to persuade her husband to get medical advice he has finally succumbed to a heart attack. She has been instrumental in getting him off to hospital or initiating some kind of treatment. The severity of his condition has been demonstrated for all to see and his survival may very probably be attributed by his nearest and dearest to the promptness with which she acted.

How can they be expected to switch, almost immediately afterwards, to an attitude which implies that caution can be thrown to the winds? It is practically inevitable that wives will continue to feel they are 'better to be safe than sorry'. The sequel to saying, 'If I hadn't got to the doctor he'd be dead' is to think, 'He must be careful, or else...' Even if they do not say it in so many words, the patient's relative is liable to dread, for some time at least, the possibility of this happening again. Like the patients, relatives will desperately seek the support of protective rituals and professional reassurance.

Severe illness does not only strike the patient. The whole family suffers. The wife of someone who has had a heart attack goes through an intensely disturbing experience. She comes up to the very verge of widowhood, she is all but bereft of her husband, almost bereaved. And just as the man may grieve and feel 'broken-hearted' because of the loss of his former picture of himself and his possibly diminished vigour, so his wife will be deeply saddened by the change she has endured. She is forced to take a fresh look at their life together and she may dread that she has in some way actually lost the strong man whom she married, even although he has 'been spared'. So she has to suffer not only the intense anxieties attendant possibly upon an emergency hospital admission and the early hours when 'anything could happen', but the sobering reflections which follow.

Suddenly life, which had been flowing easily by in a wholly predictable manner, becomes totally disorganized. No long-term plans are possible. From hour to hour over the first few days she is overwhelmed by a series of crises and changes. The whole tenor and tempo of her existence alters, kin are called in, contingency plans are made, she and others take over her husband's responsibilities. She is constantly at the bedside or visiting the hospital or phoning.

As convalescence is established she feels initial relief at having been saved from a worse fate. But her relief is short-lived and soon replaced by the special anxieties which belong to her as the main domestic guardian of her husband's physical well-being and the person whose care or carelessness could, she fancies, determine his survival or bring about his death. It is a very great responsibility for someone to bear. Small wonder that most wives in this situation tend to err on the side of caution.

There is another consideration. The patient, however worried he may feel, has at least received the reassurances of the medical and nursing staff at first hand. He is bound to have realized, whilst in hospital at least, something of current medical attitudes concerning rapid recovery and will have been started on a confident programme of progressive physical activity. If he has been in a ward he is very likely to have met and spoken with other patients, recovering from heart attacks like himself. The staff will have conveyed their firm conviction that all such patients are bound to go from strength to strength. Although the advice which is given may lack something in specificity, its tone at least will have been optimistic. All this is part of the patient's private experience of his illness and of the doctors' and nurses' judgements on him.

But the wife or other relative who is only visiting is bound to receive a very different impression of the same scene. Whilst his manifest recovery is likely to reinforce her conviction that it is the treatment he is receiving there which is 'curing' him, she will be liable to apprehension over what may happen once the doctors and nurses are no longer near.

On the other hand, if someone has been treated at home for a heart attack, his wife will have had much more responsibility for his day-to-day surveillance and care. She will have been cooperating with their own doctor and herself acting for much of the time as nurse. Whilst this responsibility may, initially, be exceedingly challenging and even alarming, as time passes and the patient is steadily recovering she will have good reason to gain confidence.

One of the key problems for any patient or their relatives faced with a new and potentially dangerous illness is that they simply do not have enough first-hand experience to give them confidence and help them make decisions on what it is safe or unwise to undertake.

Of course heart attack is so common that many people nowadays do know of a close relative or friend who has had an attack. About half of the people we interviewed, whether patients or relatives, knew of someone close to them who had suffered this way. But this does not mean that their ideas on causation or on treatment will correspond to those held currently by the medical profession. It is, for example, very widely believed that heart attacks are brought on by stress and overwork. This is, when one thinks of it, a very reassuring point of view for many people. Far from being something to be ashamed of, a heart attack is a kind of badge of courage. It is proof to one's wife and friends and work colleagues of 'overdoing it'. You have practically killed yourself with work and worry, on behalf of the family or the firm or some worthy cause. Whereas the occurrence of mental illness in a family is often carefully hidden and covered by euphemisms, heart attacks are thought of as honourable scars borne in the hard battle of life. Although the experience of a heart attack, therefore, may evoke deep personal fears about whether one's heart will 'ever be the same again', it is still a very different matter from having been diagnosed as a psychiatric case.

A person who suffers a heart attack can, at least for a time, enjoy some of the benefits of martyrdom. 'He's been overdoing it', people will say, shaking their heads in admiring disapproval. In a society where the work ethic predominates this activity is praiseworthy. Someone essentially strong-hearted and powerful has been overcome by the sheer pressure of duties and responsibilities. However, this view of heart attack causation carries the corollary that such excessive zeal should be avoided in future for fear of a recurrence.

There is also, in the popular imagination, a related and mistaken notion that heart attacks are the especial prerogative of professional men, managers and business tycoons and the like. In other words, it is still widely believed that they are commoner amongst the well-to-do who feel they have especially onerous responsibilities. This used to be the case but the position has changed and actually been reversed so that working-class or blue-collar workers are now statistically more likely to fall victim to heart attacks than are people higher up the income scale. The key risk factors are thought to be those outlined in the previous chapter, namely, smoking, high blood pressure, probably certain blood fats and a sedentary life style. These are not now the exclusive preserve of the affluent. Our general standard of living has increased over time making it likely now that all manner of men are liable to similar risks.

A further component at least of the male view regards the supposed risks which men run because of 'nagging wives'. There is no doubt that many of our own patients, when reviewing their medical history, were of the opinion that their wives were worriers, constantly fussing over the health of husbands who themselves would not condescend to such womanish fears.

But, by the time someone has actually suffered a heart attack, they are in a much weaker position. The patient may want to feel he is completely better, may want to be back to full activity and full control, but yet is secretly alarmed and depressed by the persistence of symptoms. Once they are back from hospital people very often enter on a phase of fear, frustration and sustained uncertainty. Of course individual patients inevitably differ in the manner and extent of their response to this difficult time, depending upon their own psychological make-up and the way they have previously reacted to other major life crises. At one end of the scale are the 'deniers' who sail through the experience apparently unscathed. At the opposite end are people who have severe emotional problems which persist for as long as a year after an attack.

Most people, however, come somewhere in between. Thus it is common for men to be anxious or depressed or both during the month or six weeks after an attack. It is just as well for wives and families to be forewarned about this reaction so that they can anticipate it and perhaps bear its manifestations more calmly themselves.

The person concerned is likely to be tense and irritable. They may flare up over minor frustrations and be quick to take offence at the slightest criticism. What is especially difficult for their wives to bear is that their husbands are likely to take particular exception to well-meant expressions of concern. They will object to being 'fussed over' at one moment and then seem hurt shortly after because they think their needs are not being accurately understood and catered for. They seem both dependent and resistant to dependency at the same time.

In the main, the convalescent period will simply bring out more strongly certain personality traits which were already in evidence before the attack. As I have suggested earlier, the expressions of irritation and exasperation are likely to spring from real difficulties which the patient is having with his unreliable body, which persists in providing unwelcome reminders of the recent illness, and from the worries which tend constantly to preoccupy his mind.

The situation is made worse by the fact that this is bound

to be a period of relative inactivity. Although extended bed rest is a thing of the past, the very fact of being confined to home, without a regular work routine, is liable to be exceedingly demoralizing and frustrating for many men, used to a very different way of life. The fact that they have to all intents and purposes nothing to do reduces their feeling of masculinity and, moreover, makes them more conscious of all kinds of minor bodily sensations. I said in Chapter Three that you are liable to become aware of the heart's motion if you worry about it. People who have recently had a heart attack can scarcely avoid monitoring their own heart's action and imagining it is behaving strangely, especially if they have little else to occupy their time.

It is quite common for patients to have insomnia and to be particularly concerned with their heart's present and future functioning as they lie awake and lonely whilst others are asleep. They may not, however, confess such symptoms and preoccupations to their wives or to their doctors. Thus misunderstandings multiply and often people do not ask for or receive the help they most need.

Men will not only worry about the state of their heart and the possibility of another attack. They may well brood on their sexual potential and on whether and when they can dare to resume sex. They will wonder about coping with the return to work. And, every single day, they will be faced with endless trivial decisions. 'Should I go out in this wind?' 'Can I drive the car?' 'Is this dustbin too heavy to lift?' 'Ought I to eat this?'

At the same time they find it intensely annoying and humiliating to be under perpetual surveillance by others. They resent their wives' constant supervision even whilst they may rationally accept that such concern arises from the best intentions. The fact that some of their own customary jobs around the house or garden are taken on by other family members may be felt as a mixed blessing since it is a continual reminder of their own inadequacy. Also things may not get done in the precise way they would prefer.

Meanwhile wives face severe personal difficulties as they try to persuade an unwilling spouse to conform to the picture they hold of how a heart patient should behave. As I said earlier, there are perfectly understandable reasons for the excessive caution wives usually choose to recommend. So there tends to be misunderstandings and differences on this score, about the nature and extent of all sorts of activities.

But wives may also feel themselves responsible for seeing that 'doctor's orders' are followed. Here they may encounter further resistances. For example, a patient who denies the significance and seriousness of his heart attack may get back quickly to a near normal routine. But if this includes smoking as much as before and refusing to modify his diet, his wife may feel doubly worried, both on the patient's account and because she simply cannot ensure that he will do what the doctor has said. A wife in this situation is right back in the kind of mental conflicts which we found so frequently before a heart attack had taken place.

Facing the more common combination of irritability, anxiety and depression a wife will find she is often being blamed for whatever is bothering her husband. She will be wrong when she is over-solicitous and wrong if she doesn't notice he needs her. As far as their sex life is concerned she is likely initially to repress her own desires. Indeed the resumption of relations may be far from relaxing and pleasurable as she may not be able to keep from imagining that it might perhaps kill him.

Wives depend a great deal at this particular stage on the support they get from close confidants within their own family. Friends may well supply all kinds of practical help and, to start with, the whole family will rally round. But no one takes as much of the persistent direct strain as the wife. It is she who is the butt of her husband's aggression and the source of his support. Many of her own deepest anxieties cannot be shared with him, simply because they are about him and because he is the patient whom she feels she really should be constantly sustaining and encouraging.

Men complain that they are treated differently by their families after an attack. Indeed this is inevitable. The person who has gone through such a life crisis, such a significant passage or stage, is bound to be seen differently on his return from the lonely danger. He has acquired a new identity by virtue of his momentous experience. The fact of his heart attack is something which is now an essential part of him in the eyes of others and, in the early weeks and months, may well tend to seem to his close associates the most important fact about him.

But a wife is subject to great uncertainties about the significance of any symptoms he mentions. Clearly she cannot keep summoning the doctor. After all, her husband is now officially on the mend. Nevertheless, any lay person does have great difficulty in sorting out untoward sensations and this difficulty is naturally compounded once he or she has been faced with the reality of a cardiac emergency. It is definitely not conducive to self-confidence, especially in the early stages of someone's convalescence.

The sort of problems I have mentioned in this chapter, though usually transient, are very worrying whilst they last. Many general practitioners make a point of seeing patients who have been in hospital at least within a month of returning home and they assume that virtually all of them will return to normal activities in a few months. Only the doctor who is seeing someone regularly and who can build up a complete picture of their progress can provide individual advice on the details of progressive physical activity.

But not all patients are equally fortunate in their encounters with their doctors and some feel it is a time when they could do with much more specific information and help. The kind of worries I have described may not be easy for patients and their wives to explain to doctors. Even straight physical symptoms of chest pain may be withheld. So it is not surprising if people do not express the many worries which are filling their lives but which they possibly feel cannot be conveyed to a busy practitioner in the course of a brief surgery appointment. Even six months after an attack many patients and their famiies may still be confused over what kinds of activities are possible or advisable. Sexual difficulties may be particularly hard to bring out during a routine 'physical' follow-up and, even if they are aired, may be lamentably one-sided if the partner is not brought into the picture.

People who are passing through such a significant transition period in their lives do need confident professional support. They definitely require clear, specific guidelines to hold on to and prefer to be given positive instructions about graded exercise, about details of diet and about whether they should modify their sexual and social activities. Concrete instructions are called for, not vague statements of encouragement or veiled caution. Patients really need the precise nature of their jobs to be assessed, in terms of what they involve in both physical and emotional strain. Advice at this stage simply has to be individualized because each person is facing or anticipating unique problems.

Some people are fortunate in being able to modify their lives without too much conflict and unhappiness. Indeed it is possible that a time for reflection such as this may change a person's view on what is most important and valuable in his life. He takes stock and sorts out what gives him most satisfaction and what activities he can thankfully cut down or eliminate in future. Some husbands, obliged to stay at home for some weeks whilst their wives are out at work, may find that taking over some of their roles is positively congenial.

But not many are so fortunate, either because of the nature of their work, which simply does not permit of modification, or because they cannot become reconciled to the constant arguments and differences within the family.

It is abundantly clear that psychological and social factors are just as important as medical ones in determining when a person gets back to work. Some American psychiatrists feel strongly that physical exercise is the best means of combating depression and they routinely prescribe a special course of training. But not every doctor is convinced of the necessity to concentrate on this one aspect of physical fitness. Regular exercise is certainly to be encouraged, both in healthy individuals and in cardiac patients. The form it takes must be for the patient and his doctor to decide. Sometimes there are programmes of supervised exercise training available in special centres. Others may prefer cycling, jogging or games.

The benefits to someone's morale can be very considerable. But the exercise should be enjoyable in its own right, otherwise people will soon drop out of a programme. Patients should not be forced to take part in exercise; it should be freely chosen because it is seen as contributing to their optimum efficiency and sense of well-being.

An important source of help during rehabilitation comes from other people in the same situation. Self-help groups for heart attack patients and their wives have sprung up in many parts of America but are not yet common in Britain. People derive tremendous satisfaction from sharing their experiences and problems. They find that others who have had a heart attack are willing listeners who can identify easily with the drama of the original event and the multiple dilemmas of rehabilitation. Comparing and finding differences between their own symptoms, treatment regimes and reactions and those of other survivors is a source of real support. They can also swop stories about the tedium of constant supervision by their wives and other members of the family. Groups like these are often helped by the presence of a nurse or someone with professional knowledge, short of a medical training. They need to feel free to express their criticisms of doctors as well as their deep dependence on them and to be helped decide what problems and symptoms are worth taking for medical help.

Whilst many male patients who have experienced these groups agree that their wives too could benefit from them, they would prefer the two sorts of meeting to be separate. That way more openness is possible and self-confidence is enhanced. The mere knowledge that others have been dealing with problems as bad as your own private ones can be a great source of relief. People can share their solutions as well as their difficulties and begin to see the positive gains which can come from more knowledge of themselves and their partners. A remarkable sense of cohesion and loyalty can arise in groups like these.

6
Prevention

'Can I avoid a heart attack?' was the anxious title of an article in the *Lancet* a few years ago. It expressed the universal human desire to escape serious misfortune and was at the same time the kind of specific question people regularly put to their doctors. No one wants to be ill. But the full impact is only appreciated by people who have experienced it. Hence the urge towards prevention is likely to be particularly strong among those who have already had one heart attack, but it also motivates people who are aware of its effect on someone close to them.

As men reach middle age they begin anxiously to scan the health record of their contemporaries. Most can name a workmate or acquaintance who has had a heart attack. Some of those will even have been heard to boast, 'I've had my first heart attack', thereby demonstrating their own personal capacity for survival whilst confessing the constant fear of a recurrence.

Any severe illness, carrying the threat of death or some degree of disability, makes us ask questions. 'Why has this happened to me? Why just at this time? Whatever can I have done to deserve it?' Later, as the worst is over, the demand comes for help to avoid having to go through the same experience again.

Doctors may not be good at answering fundamental questions about the particularity of human misfortune. But they have been trained to follow chains of physical causation as explanations for the manifestations of disease. They are also well accustomed to providing prescriptions for behaviour at the same time as dealing out drugs. So they are keen to supply patients and potential patients with advice on this very important contemporary disease.

There is absolutely no doubt about patients' need for reassuring advice and doctors' desire to provide it. The problem lies in the continuing state of uncertainty regarding the disease process itself. This is certainly not for lack of research. The subject has generated a vast amount of investigation throughout the Western world but, in spite of all this activity, the results are still inconclusive.

The subject was considered in Chapter Four and I shall do no more than summarize it again here. Blood cholesterol levels are lower in poor than in affluent communities and, broadly, it is the latter which are most liable to have ischaemic heart disease. Moreover, there is a close association between the proportion of total calories taken in the form of saturated fats and the cholesterol in the blood.

However, it has not yet been convincingly demonstrated within groups which are at high risk of developing ischaemic heart disease that there is a direct association between an individual's fat intake and that individual's cholesterol levels.

Changing diets experimentally in groups of people who are in institutional care by strictly limiting the amount and nature of their fats can bring down the overall level of blood cholesterol. Such diets are very rigorous, resembling, as far as fat content is concerned, that of the poor communities who experience few heart attacks. It is difficult to persuade ordinary healthy people to stick to such meals voluntarily for the long period necessary to discern results in terms of changes in death rates from heart disease, and there is disturbing evidence that deaths from other causes may actually be increased in the process.

But the great bulk of any population, whatever their blood cholesterol, will not develop ischaemic heart disease. For instance, a man of forty-five with a blood cholesterol of 210 milligrams per 100 millilitres of blood and who is a non-smoker, with normal blood pressure, has about a one-in-eight chance of developing ischaemic heart disease in the next twenty years. His friend, whose characteristics are similar but whose cholesterol is 310 mg/100 ml, has just over a one-in-five risk throughout the same future. The risk attributable directly to raised cholesterol is only 4.3 per cent over a period of twenty years. In other words, the amount of risk attributable to raised blood cholesterol is still relatively small. Even where cholesterol levels exceed 300 mg the numbers of men who do not develop ischaemic heart disease in the next ten or twenty years greatly exceed those who do.

Is it justifiable to embark upon a concerted effort to change dietary fat intakes? Will people who are without any symptoms be prepared to change to an unpalatable diet and keep it up for many years on the chance that substantially lowering their blood cholesterol may reduce the risk that some of them will have a coronary?

It should be remembered too that there is not a one-to-one relationship between ischaemic heart disease and atheroma in the arteries. Although most of those who develop heart attacks have atheroma the contrary is certainly not the case.

Long before the present epidemic of ischaemic heart disease, 30 per cent of men dying from other causes had advanced atheroma of their coronary arteries. These two conditions do not correspond to one another therefore, even though they often overlap.

A clear predictor of heart attacks is a history of angina, the history of a possible previous infarct or suggestive signs on an electro-cardiogram. These are all relatively easy to determine.

If someone is in this category their prospects are better if they have low levels of blood cholesterol and a low blood pressure, if they are not overweight and if they do not smoke cigarettes. But it does not follow that the higher risk of people who have less favourable characteristics, who smoke or have a raised blood cholesterol for instance, will necessarily be improved by advice or by treatment.

You should not be unduly alarmed by the mention of angina as a warning symptom. The great majority of people who have angina will not go on to develop heart attacks. Even in the highest risk categories, men who are older and have a history or signs of a previous possible heart attack, less than 10 per cent will die of ischaemic heart disease in the next ten years.

So there are several persisting areas of uncertainty. The first is the absence of a direct relationship between someone's fat intake and his own blood cholesterol level. The second is the impossibility of saying, even at a high level of this particular 'risk factor', whether a specific person is going to have a heart attack. The third grey area has to do with the fact that it has not yet been proved that reduction of unfavourable characteristics (blood pressure, blood cholesterol, weight, smoking) will improve the prognosis and reduce the risk for someone who already has evidence of ischaemic heart disease, in the form of symptoms of angina or a previous scar on the heart.

Meanwhile there are some encouraging new developments. Deaths from heart attacks are now falling in the United States. In 1978 they had dropped below the one million per year mark. At the same time there has been a decline in mortality from all causes, but the size of the drop in deaths from coronaries has been the largest.

There is no doubt that Americans have lately become increasingly responsive to advice about diet and smoking and exercise. Many cardiologists in the United States do not hesitate to attribute the lowered death rates to these changes in life style. They have been much readier than their British counterparts to believe that there is a direct connection between dietary fats and ischaemic heart disease. It is the reduction of dietary fats that is recommended above all, by authoritative organizations in America and New Zealand, for instance. Indeed in some circles it is almost heretical to question this dogma.

But some powerful dissenting voices are nevertheless raised. The opponents of what they call 'the diet heart hypothesis' point out that the quantity of polyunsaturated fats, which are supposedly the answer to heart attacks, consumed in the United States have doubled since 1900. During the same time there has been little or no change in the amount of saturated fats or cholesterol which has been eaten. This period covers the development of the heart disease epidemic which we have been experiencing. Such critics attribute the recently improving death rates from the disease to better coronary care or to changes in aspects of life apart from diet, such as more vigorous exercise – in the form of jogging, for instance – or giving up smoking.

British opinion is on the whole still guarded. The report on Diet and Coronary Disease published by the Department of Health and Social Security declared that no single item in the diet could be implicated and, furthermore, that it had not been proved that reducing blood cholesterol lessened the risk of developing heart attacks. But they did note with concern a recent rise in the overall proportion of fat in the British diet. So they recommended that fat intake should be reduced, especially animal, saturated fats. However, they did not go to the length of advocating more polyunsaturated fats. They did point out that it was desirable to avoid obesity. In fact the recommendations of these doctors amount to advocating moderation in all things. Since then spokesmen for the Royal College of Physicians and the British Cardiac Society have reviewed all the research to date. They ended by cautiously saying it would be advisable partially to substitute unsaturated fats for saturated, animal fats. In addition they recommended the general reduction of fat in the diet.

One of the most recent developments has been the suggestion, from research in Britain, that a high fibre diet may be protective. These studies, followed up over twenty years among civil service staff and bus drivers and conductors, showed a lower incidence of ischaemic heart disease in men who had a high intake of dietary fibre from cereals at the time the survey began. Smoking was a further, independent factor influencing the likelihood of heart attacks. People with a high energy intake were the healthiest. This is closely related to physical activity, so the importance of exercise is once more in the forefront of the picture.

Moderate alcohol consumption may actually be protective

too. It seems that alcohol may increase the level of certain 'high density lipoproteins' which have been shown to be associated with lower heart attack risks. But excessive alcohol can damage the heart muscle. Currently research is focusing upon naturally occurring substances in the blood, called prostaglandins, which are probably of key importance in affecting blood clotting.

What does all this amount to for the ordinary patient or the person who is worried that he might someday have a heart attack? It is clear that the experts disagree on details. But the advantages of reducing weight are not in doubt. Whilst this can be achieved in several different ways, it would be prudent to reduce the amount of fat and sugar that are consumed.

You may, if you wish, partly substitute margarine for butter. But, if you decide to conform to a diet low in saturated fats, avoid coconut oil. The vegetable oils to choose are corn oil, soya bean oil or, preferably, sunflower seed oil. It is important to try to discover what are the precise vegetable oils used in prepared food stuffs. We eat a great deal of commercially processed foods these days but it is exceedingly difficult to be sure what they contain. Do not use the same cooking fat repeatedly, reheating time and again. There is a danger that cancer-causing oxidized substances could be formed.

You may well find it worthwhile to move to a diet containing more cereals and rough fibres. It has already been shown to aid many digestive conditions. Now it looks as though it might protect you against heart disease.

Cigarette smoking should be stopped. It is easy to advise this, less easy to achieve. But there is little doubt of its harmful effects on the cardiac circulation. Pipe and cigar smoking, because the smoke is not inhaled, carry considerably less danger.

Exercise certainly makes you feel better. It takes an effort to begin, especially if you have not been in the habit of taking regular exercise. Evidence is building up that we should all take a lot more exercise – the more vigorous the better. But be advised on the details by your own doctor. A graduated programme is what is needed, not a wild rush to break former, youthful records.

The question of raised blood pressure is one for a physician to determine. There are now potent drugs available which will reduce hypertension. But they generally need to be taken for a prolonged period. Some have unpleasant side effects about which your doctor should be kept informed.

The suggestions are none of them extreme. Perhaps some people would feel safer with exceedingly rigid rules, but there is no guarantee that they would ward off danger. It is best to take comfort in the fact that your chances of not having a heart attack far exceed the chances of becoming a victim. Meanwhile the best advice is to avoid excesses of food or slothfulness, prudent measures which have been recommended by physicians since Hippocrates' day.

A woman's diary

I shall now share with you extracts from my diary over a period of two months in 1977 when my husband was developing a cardiac illness which eventually came to need open-heart surgery. Although his was not a heart attack, the events of these months were fraught with uncertainty for our whole family and their fundamentally puzzling and disturbing nature was not noticeably eased by the fact that I myself was a physician.

John was the Labour Member of Parliament for a constituency close to Edinburgh. Our children, Deirdre and Stuart, who were then seven and nine, lived at home as did my teenage son, Tunde, the youngest child of my previous marriage. My other children were both in their twenties, Paul working in England and Aysha then a medical student in Wales. My stepdaughter Charlotte and her brother Malcolm, in their late teens, visited us frequently. We were, I suppose, an unusually large but close family.

The story begins in midsummer.

Wednesday 22 June:

Just back from examining at Leeds University. This is the busiest time of the entire academic year. Our own students' exams next. Deirdre is getting so excited about the camping holiday. It's two years since we've been to France. Foolishly we decided to stay at home in '76. So the joy of anticipation is specially great now. Every night that he's at home at a weekend Deirdre climbs up on her father's knee after the meal and says, 'Now tell me *exactly* what the holiday will be like?' I find myself being quite unreasonably irritated. I suppose it's because she seems to be monopolizing the very limited time and attention John can spare us.

Saturday 25 June:

Up at the crack of dawn to drive Tunde to Prestwick. Aysha arrives on vacation this afternoon. Have my inoculations for forthcoming trip to Nigeria as external examiner. There is an unsettling feeling of too much travelling and people moving here and there. I don't like it.

Tuesday 28 June:

Deirdre is recovering from a stomach upset, she's had thirty-six hours of vomiting and fever.

This afternoon John spent working to replace the glass panels in the shower. It is an awkward job. He is tired and irritable. Malcolm is visiting and was enlisted to help.

About 6 John comes into the kitchen looking very exhausted.

'I think I'm having a heart attack...' he says. I answer 'Rubbish... go and wash and come for supper... you're just tired.'

Over supper Malcolm is chatting to him. Asks a question.

He can't reply. He is very pale and pinched looking. I see that he may really be ill. He goes to lie down upstairs. I deliberately wait for twenty minutes to allow him to become composed and also because I don't want to panic everyone. When I do go up to see him he just seems very tired.

Wednesday 29 June:
After a very restless night (he's had bad nights for weeks...) John has gone through to the bed in my study. I prepare a breakfast-tray and carry it in. He sits up. As he does so he suddenly becomes pale, sweating, vomits. I take his pulse, it's weak, low volume. He says he has epigastric pain. I'm sure it's a heart attack.

Tell him to stay lying down. Show no alarm. Calm him. Get out of the room and immediately tell Aysha what I think is happening. Tell her to go in to him whilst I phone the doctor. Make my diagnosis clear to the receptionist, remind her I'm a doctor so I know what I'm talking about.

Senior partner is round in 10-15 minutes. I describe what I call 'cardiogenic shock'. He orders John to the Accident and Emergency Department by ambulance. He is taken off without pyjamas or slippers.

I jump in my little Citröen and follow. As I drive I'm mentally preparing myself to be 'the wife of a heart attack victim'.

Wait in Accident and Emergency for what seems ages.

'Look, the ECG is OK,' says the resident doctor triumphantly, allowing me as a physician to view the tracing. John is still on a trolley. He looks no better... But the test has decided otherwise. So he's transferred to a chair for the long corridor trip to the X-ray department, where I wait again.

'Look, the X-ray's OK too,' the same Accident and

Emergency doctor is delighted to announce. 'It's probably just gastroenteritis... or perhaps, pancreatitis...'

I help John back into the car under a blanket and set off home. As my own serious diagnosis hasn't been confirmed I feel less pressed. So I stop at the butcher's.

When I come out John is mortified because of an old lady's astonishment as she peered into the parked car and saw him, draped only in a blanket, vomiting miserably.

Although the episode in the Accident and Emergency was so cursory it has been very reassuring to him. He's always been worried about his heart, even long before we first met. I diagnosed 'cardiac neurosis' and made fun of his fears.

Friday 1 July:
The doctor hasn't been back. I think John is slowly but perceptibly recovering. He's still very restless at night and his breath is bad. It must have been his stomach. Today I've been ill and exhausted myself. I've spent the whole day in bed. That makes three of us who've had the same bug. Rather surprisingly John sits for a lot of the afternoon in the bedroom with me. He talks of nothing but his own symptoms.

Saturday 2 July:
Help John in the garden.

Sunday 3 July:
My birthday. The children run in with gifts. I spend the morning 'slaving in the kitchen'. John watches his own Granada programme on TV. Then he dresses extra carefully so as to prove he is better and we go out for our pre-lunch drink. As we leave the house I enquire, rather sarcastically,

whether he'd like me to drive today, knowing full well what the answer will be. John takes tomato juice today.

Monday 4 July:
John is vomiting again. Feels weakness too. He is very surprised and disappointed by this setback. Resentful of enforced invalidism. Nothing very definite that I can sort out. The pain has shifted from his epigastrium. It's more over the liver now. (I forgot to say the doctor had found it enlarged last week.)

At night I notice that whereas I, who have recently embarked on a somewhat erratic course of 'relaxation' through controlled respiration, breathe twelve to the minute at rest, John, asleep, is breathing twenty-four to the minute. Surely that is wrong?

He's still fussing about his heart. He says his pulse rate is increased – as indeed it is. Says he 'hasn't lost weight, though hardly eating all week'. The other day he came off the bathroom scales announcing he'd actually gained two pounds. I just don't believe it...

A few weeks ago I noted that, though he has improved his chest and arm muscles through systematic weight lifting recently, he seems to have developed a curious bulge in his epigastrium. Liver perhaps?

Tuesday 5 July:
John is much weaker today. I call the surgery by noon.

'No. It isn't an emergency this time... but he's not recovering as he should... I want Dr Graham to call.'

He stays in bed most of the day then dresses slowly and comes cautiously downstairs to sit with me in the late afternoon sun at the front door, where Dr Graham presently finds us. The GP embarks on what is, essentially, social chat.

At length John precedes the doctor, very slowly, upstairs. 'Did Dr Graham notice how short of breath he is?' I wonder. The doctor decides he's convalescing.

This evening John reluctantly agrees that I should deputize for him at the opening of a Church sale tomorrow. I say I can manage it, after a morning meeting of my own. I'll take the kids.

Wednesday 6 July:

I felt so much in need of a proper night's sleep I went through to the study. This morning I was surprised to hear John going downstairs to the postman first thing and, shortly after, arranging over the phone to do the constituency engagement himself. His voice sounds perfectly confident and normal.

I enter the bedroom.

'So you don't want me to speak at Dunbar?'

'No. I'm better.'

'But at least I'll come with you?'

'You won't have time, I'm leaving at noon.'

I feel rejected, my best intentions cast aside. I also worry about him taking Deirdre, who is still keen to go. I think, 'Even if John feels he's a little better he could well collapse in the car. Though I can't stop my husband from going, at least I can stop my child from being at risk.' So I dissuade her from accompanying her father.

He returns in the late evening, very tired indeed, and goes straight to bed.

During these last few days I've phoned two people for support and advice. Alex [a Nigerian doctor friend] says, 'Get him into the coronary care unit... Cut through all the intervening people.' Colin [his radiologist brother in London] says, 'Call in a friendly cardiologist to reassure him about his heart... he's always had a cardiac neurosis... I'll see him myself when next he's down in London.'

I do neither. He is, after all, seeming better... I don't want to go against, or behind, the GP... Anyway, I can't decide which consultant would be appropriate...

Friday 8 July:
Can I still go to Nigeria? Should I go to Nigeria? It's only for the weekend, a few days...

Charlotte says, 'Go – I'll cope. The Old Man is just fussing...'

John meanwhile is out to lunch anyway, so he can't be too bad.

By 4.30 he's not back. It is the last moment, I shall have to drive myself to the airport. I leave a brief farewell note on his study table, affectionate, concerned.

Our cars meet in the drive. I don't get out. He is pale and tense.

'Can you... will you drive me to the airport?' I ask.

'I'm too tired.'

'Whatever have you been doing all this time?' I feel cross after being worried.

'Buying the weekend food,' he replies wearily.

'Why ever do it on a Friday afternoon?' I ask and drive off feeling irritated.

When I phone home from Heathrow he sounds cheerful, domesticated and paternal. I reckon he's found my note.

In the air I write to a friend in America about the events of the last few days, 'there's a strong psychosomatic element, I suspect'.

Tuesday 12 July:

Home from Africa at 10 p.m. 'Where is John?' I ask my stepdaughter. 'Gone down to London...but he says he'll return tomorrow.'

'How has he been, then?'

'Fussing about being tired.'

'Has he prepared the car for camping?'

'Not yet – there wasn't time.'

Wednesday 13 July:

My work colleagues are amused at the idea of going to Nigeria for a weekend.

9.30 p.m.: John is still not back. Stuart and I are alone together in the upstairs sitting-room. Deirdre is in her bath.

I hear a sound, like a faint cry in the hall. But we haven't heard the car arrive. And no one appears. Decide it couldn't be John.

10 minutes pass.

John glides into the room – a ghost, trembling, cold, shocked. Been sick at Heathrow, again at Turnhouse airport, declined a doctor's offer of a lift, drove home, couldn't make it up the stairs, had lain down in his study...

We get him warmed up on the couch before the fire. He revives.

He tells how he called his brother in London who arranged for a full cardiac check-up at a London hospital. 'Absolutely nothing the matter with his heart.' But he'd had such difficulty trying to keep pace with his brother walking along a short incline... Someone at the airport said, 'How are you?' He replied, 'I feel absolutely dreadful, like death.' But the other didn't seem to notice his words, the enquiry had been purely routine.

Thursday 14 July:
An Irish academic colleague is visiting, for lunch. John comes gingerly downstairs. Later he emerges to sit in a deck chair in the sunny garden. He jokes about his weak condition.

I notice how very distended his stomach looks now, seated at that angle. Like a pregnancy almost. It must be fluid, I'm sure.

My sister Sheila turns up. I take her aside into the house. Tell her how desperately worried I am about John. I just cannot believe he means to drive us all off on a camping holiday in two days. The idea must be quashed.

So far the children have no idea that anything is amiss.

John excuses himself to go back indoors and write a newspaper article. Afterwards up to bed. His colleague apologizes profusely for calling at a difficult time. But John assures him it is nothing, we are about to leave for the South of France.

Friday 15 July:
John even weaker this morning. For the third time I summon the GP. When he arrives I convince him of my worry and puzzlement. He doesn't seem to take much notice of the abdominal distension and my idea of retained fluid...

He decides to involve a second opinion. A specialist in infectious diseases. As he speaks to his colleague over the phone I fidget round the study, flicking at furniture with a duster.

I am to drive John at once to the former Fever Hospital.

I go upstairs and start preparing to leave. John is in tears.

'Why am I so much weaker today?' He can't really get ready. Decides he must bathe. Is barely capable of struggling back to the bedroom. Collapses wet and naked on the bed. I proffer a dressing-gown and either new pyjamas or a suit. Chooses the suit. 'Do I need a tie?' (He's usually so particular about his ties.) Almost too weak to dress at all.

Comes down the stairs, unaided but *in extremis*. My car is at the front door. Falls back into the passenger seat. He doesn't respond to conversation. His eyes are closed. He objects to the draught from the open window.

It is a beautiful summer's day. The front gardens are full of roses. He sees none of it.

At the entrance to the ward there is no one to be seen. I search desperately for a wheelchair. John looks barely conscious in the lonely parked car... Find a resident who gets a staff nurse to bring a chair and 'jollies him along' towards bed.

He says we can keep his silver cuff links when he's dead.

Settled in bed against high pillows with all his few personal possessions itemized and sorted. He is breathing very fast.

I rush home to feed the children. Return in the late afternoon with Deirdre and Stuart in tow. We begin an anxious evening, commuting between a vantage point just within the ward corridor, from which we can see doctors round their Dad's bed, and the visitors' room.

We are told we can if we wish 'spend the night'. A clear warning of doom. Deirdre senses it and objects. But Stuart is prepared to settle down to enjoy the lounge facilities.

I am summoned alone to hear the consultant's diagnosis: 'Coxsackie myocarditis and pericarditis' [a virus infection of the heart muscle and its outer covering]. I feel quite absurdly pleased by the final clever 'naming' of what has so long been obscure or denied. Only later do I realize its implications... There is no treatment.

I take the children home, via a fish and chip shop. Now they both know the holidays will be 'put off for a week'. Deirdre immediately starts listing alternative entertainments. Her brother is more realistic and solemn about the so-called 'postponement'.

Once home I call Sheila and a radiologist in Canada. He says 'Don't lose hope...'

Late at night Paul [my eldest son] arrives unexpectedly. A most welcome surprise. We talk till 2 a.m.

Saturday 16 July:

My sister arrives by car from England. My son Tunde is back this morning from Canada but I can't spare even a moment to speak to him.

All day at the hospital. John is clearly in cardiac and liver failure. His colour is florid, with a shade of jaundice. The slightest movement makes him breathless. His hand against his cheek is pale, it looks so like my dead father's hand. I sit very close and talk to him when it seems he can hear.

Leave him briefly in the afternoon. When I return, only two hours later, he is very restless and distressed. 'It's so kind of you to come back,' he whispers.

He is worse. More anxious and fearful of dying now.

Very late at night I return home, to find the sitting-room full of extended family, my own and my sister's. They are all talking and laughing and drinking beer. It seems blasphemous to me, they do not sense the horror. The talk is trivial. No one knows or respects my anguish.

I make a series of phone calls. Harry, a doctor friend, arrives. His intense seriousness about John's condition (he called at the hospital this afternoon) makes me even more nervous.

Sunday 17 July:
John even worse. I stay all day. In the afternoon he has a definite cyanotic attack, becomes very blue. I summon the house physician and tell her. But will she pass on the message?

'When is the cardiologist going to see him?' I demand to know.

Etiquette must be followed. It is, after all, the weekend. The Registrar, when told, will possibly alert the consultant who may in turn call the cardiologist if necessary.

I shall spend the entire night by John's side. I sit by him till 6 a.m. He has several more attacks of restless panic and fear of death.

I cannot see his colour now in the darkness.

There are only two other nursing attendants on the entire ward besides me. I am the cardiac monitor...

At 6 a.m. I go for a couple of hours' rest in the 'visitors' suite'. I'm wakened by the phone at 9 a.m. to say my sister is returning home. Does she think it was a false alarm? Is he taking too long to die? Paul, my eldest, is leaving today too. I remember Jesus in the Garden of Gethsemane, saying 'Will ye not wait with me even one hour?'

Monday 18 July:
Back with John. The consultant does not appear until 12.30. His first words with me are solemn and avuncular. He shows me the unhelpful X-rays. But presently he does spot something new. It may be a collection of fluid round the heart.

He calls the cardiologist, who appears within ten minutes.

Sudden emergency action. Oxygen is ordered. There is to be a transfer to the main hospital.

I grab John's few things and cram them in a plastic bag, under my arm. I carry one red rose, in a slim vase, in my other hand as I sit in the ambulance. It stops at every traffic light.

When we reach the hospital it is raining. We have to wait for a trolley.

Into the coronary care unit, site of my research of two years ago. I try with next to nothing to convert this tiny temporary cubicle into a safe home. Set up the rose, clock, pictures crayonned by the children.

An echocardiogram is connected to John. There seems like a crowd around the bed. Tense discussion. Conclusion, 'It is ambiguous, due to "interference" . . . '

The decision is made for an exploratory operation, a thoracotomy [opening the chest]. At once.

So soon is the small CCU nest destroyed.

I'd reassured John, alarmed at the sudden move; 'No one ever dies in the CCU.'

He is wheeled out, away, upstairs. I feel I am watching him go for the last time. Say casually, 'Okay then, I'll see you soon . . . '

The cardiologist told me I could wait down in the CCU. But when I come back from the outside corridor an ugly nurse is in the empty nest. She has another plastic bag.

'Can I have a list of your husband's possessions?'

I rebel. Snatch up all his few pathetic things and bundle them into my own handbag and shopper. The black striped vase has lost all its water on the ambulance trip. The rose hangs limply out of it.

With what calm I can muster I leave the ward, where I am now clearly out of place.

I cross to the empty, Sunday office. Another familiar

place, in what seems like a previous incarnation. I pace about. 'So this is it... I'm a widow – or a near as makes no difference. OK, so how do I tell the kids?'

I pick up the phone to tell my friend, a doctor's wife. 'I think I can cope, but I just can't be sure.' She will come at once...

We go together, quite slowly, across the car park and up to Ward 17. Harry, her husband, is there before us.

The cardiologist and Sister explain the position.

Charlotte joins us in Sister's room.

I know John is being prepared for surgery.

Suddenly I feel very hungry. It seems absurd, wrong, but I can't help it. My friends will take me to an Italian restaurant whilst the operation is done.

I am allowed in to see John. 'So you're all going to a party? I wish I could join you,' he says to me. I kick myself for saying we are going out for a meal.

He asks his friend, 'What do you think? They say they'll have to operate... I don't trust them...'

When we return Harry says he thinks the cardiologist is looking cheerful. He is wrong, the diagnosis was incorrect. The operation has failed to reveal any fluid which might have been burdening the heart.

I can see John now. Back from theatre. In intensive care. Not a pretty sight. On a respirator, stripped, tubes everywhere.

The doctors say, 'If we haven't done him any good at least we've done him no harm.'

But to me, suddenly become non-medical, he looks very much worse because now he's unconscious and intubated. Lost to me.

I want to stay. All the time till now I've helped him

through the worst. I think, irrationally, 'Suppose he wakes, in terror and alone.' I feel that by consenting to surgery I have simply condemned him to a painful death.

I am prevailed upon to return home. The kids are still up. In even such a small way it is relaxing to discover 'normal' life still going on at home (a feature of each short foray from hospitals these past several long, long days).

Tuesday 19 July:
Wake at 5 a.m. to see clearly, in my mind's eye, John's tortured form, rigid, intubated...

And he'd always had a 'cardiac neurosis', always dreaded hospitals, always been sure he'd die if 'they' got hold of him 'in there'.

It all seems such a waste. He's only forty-seven.

The children have said how they miss 'his funny stories at suppertime'. They've been colouring cards for him, not knowing he's past looking at them.

The next day, when John seemed all but dead, he was taken to the operating theatre again. This time open-heart surgery was performed and what appeared to be a large, simple tumour which had been blocking the inside of one chamber was successfully removed. His life had been saved, at the eleventh hour.

I now give some further extracts, from the convalescence period:

Friday 22 July:
I am not surprised to be requested to come, at 4 p.m., to see John's doctors in private. Think it must be about the detailed management of his convalescence.

I'm wearing a bright summer outfit, with a bunch of flowers pinned on my lapel. I feel restored. Sit relaxed and calm in a little-used attic study above the ward awaiting the arrival of the cardiologist and surgeon.

Then they tell me: 'It's not a simple, benign tumour but a sarcoma [malignant]. No one knows what will happen... seems to have been completely removed...but could recur at any time... Should we tell your husband?'

I am surprised to find myself hesitating... I've always taught my students, for years, that patients have 'the right to know'... but it seems such a terrible shame...

We go down together to the ward. I enter first. The surgeon 'explains'.

John says, 'Do you mean it's cancer? I didn't know you could get cancer of the *heart*.' [Tumours of the heart are in fact exceedingly rare.]

He looks pale, drawn, his lips tight. He thanks them politely.

After they've gone his head falls back on the pillow. We discuss, briefly. He is optimistic, emphasizing the positive, seems unperturbed. (The beginning of 'denial'?)

I am devastated. Thrown right back to Square One.

Sunday 24 July:
The children return from their brief token holiday with Sheila and Charlotte. We drive straight from the station to the ward.

John has been extremely tense, dissatisfied, frustrated these past few days. Irritated by sundry minor restrictions. Can't wait to get out.

The children are very subdued. It's their first sight of their father since his admission to hospital.

John tries to take Deirdre on his knee. She shrinks away. He shows them his huge chest wounds. (I'd warned him the day before not to do so.)

Deirdre is noticeably alarmed.

Monday 25 July:
This evening Deirdre is desperately upset, weeping inconsolably. She insists that we have a private talk in her bedroom. It is difficult as Stuart is jealous of our intimacy and keeps noisily interrupting.

Deirdre tells me how frightened she is. How she fears she will die if she falls asleep. How she feels she is split into two halves, her good half is her left side, the side of the thumb she sucks, the other half is bad. She is afraid of the bad side taking over. All the while she is clinging to me, terribly agitated.

By this time Stuart is incensed, upset, indignant... It is impossible to reason with him... He totally misinterprets my reasons for taking time to comfort Deirdre. She has sworn me to tell no one else about her fears.

But I do mention it later to the older ones, Tunde and Charlotte, so as to explain to them how a parent's illness can affect a small child, and to make them tolerant of Stuart's behaviour too. He is very cross and rude and short-tempered. No doubt he is resenting the limitations brought by his father's illness. But he won't say so. He has to try to seem sympathetic and mature.

Tuesday 26 July:
Pick up John from hospital. When he comes down from the ward with Charlotte and the Sister, and I look across from where my car was parked, I don't recognize him for a

moment. He looks astonishingly frail, pale and shrunken.

At home, he walks slowly around his beloved garden with great appreciation.

Thursday 28 July:
Whilst I am out to post a mass of 'thank you for get well greetings' letters I drop into my workplace to glance at my own cold mail in the bleak office.

Absolutely horrified on my return home to find John had driven the car while I was away.

I realize I might have avoided this danger if I'd either refused to go out to the post or come straight back.

John, who has been complaining all week of my continually 'persecuting' him by my precautions, at last begins to see, through my distress, just what is motivating me... From this point he begins to recognize what Charlotte and I have been engaged on over these past days and weeks... There are still big periods of his illness about which he has no personal recollection...

He tells us of the terrible cardiac nightmares at the time of the operation. Charlotte and I reconstruct for him parts of our joint past, our worst fears that he would die and our relief at the miraculous operation.

Monday 1 August:
John is very labile these days and expresses emotion much more easily than before. He is openly very grateful for my care and attention now. He weeps at the first meeting with one close friend. And again, when his brother visits.

Facially John looks tremulous and strained, like his long-dead mother these days, whilst his younger brother is the picture of health.

Thursday 4 August:
In this, the second week of John's return home, in bright and beautiful weather, we've 'come out' officially to the Press and radio, that is to say we publicly announce his progressive improvement and gratitude for an entirely successful operation.

Having done so I myself feel more positive, almost safe. It is like a '*rite de passage*', with a transitional stage past, the darkness seems to be over.

I send for my files from the office and start sorting correspondence.

Saturday 6 August:
John buys a paddling pool for the kids. He is delighted because the shop assistant spoke as if he didn't know he'd been ill.

Thursday 11 August:
A routine visit to hospital for a check-up. X-ray first. The consultant tells us all is fine.

In fact John does look well, we've been planning a holiday together. His step is jaunty. He sits down outside the doctor's room of the cardiac ward, with *The Times* under his arm, chatting confidently to another reporting-back convalescent.

I wait by the corridor window, reading a *New Society* article on 'Doctors and Death'. Could have written it myself, just my (academic) line!

John approaches. I rise to join him.

He is devastated, broken, defeated. Has been told, 'Wound infected... may need another op...complications...wait meantime for your own surgeon to come out of theatre . . .'

I jump to the secret, wild, worst conclusion, that 'infection' is merely a euphemism. Begin to anticipate the end . . . Envisage the swollen scar (just beneath his fancy ties he liked so much, used constantly to finger) as a portion of spreading malignant tissue. Think of the horror of recurrence in women with breast cancer . . .

The holiday, the whole future, all gone . . . The 'brave face on things' . . . the thank you letters gone out . . . the 'business as usual' message to the Press . . . I think I must get 'permission' for him to be nursed terminally at home.

We go out for coffee while waiting. I catch a glimpse of a colleague who eyes us quizzically. He must be thinking, 'It's fine to be some people . . . on compassionate leave right through August, both of them bronzed and well.'

A series of small further operations followed, to deal with persistent infection. During this period John was very labile, depressed and irritable, physically wasted, in frequent pain and emotionally drained. He was easily exhausted by well-meaning but uncomprehending visitors. Towards the end of August he had begun to pick up.

Wednesday 24 August:
John's forty-eighth birthday. Charlotte lets Stuart help her with a big baking for tea. I can hear him singing as he goes about his task!

The poor little boy's life has so changed these days. He gets virtually no special attention, yet he's expected to behave well, keep quiet and is rebuked when he's noisy and rude. Sometimes he's become very abusive towards John.

He has slammed the study door so hard that the knob is loose.

Tunde can also be riled these days by the endless emphasis on John's illness.

Charlotte and I are closer than we've ever been.

I'm absolutely determined to have a big family photograph today. Everyone is here except Malcolm who is in Morocco now after the alarm of failing to meet up with us at the appointed French campsite.

All eight of us assemble, specially dressed up for the occasion. It is getting dark, definitely autumn now, but the room is bright and warm. A jolly scene, lots of chaff and amusement. We dispose ourselves around the sofa for the snap.

When the film fails to develop properly in our dark-room I become almost hysterical.

During the following year John managed, with total success, to 'deny' the diagnosis and achieved more in his career than ever before.

In July 1978, after a brief illness which, in its stealth and mystery, almost mirrored the past, he was bluntly told that the tumour had regrown, uncontrollably.

'This is the unhappiest day of my life,' he said. And, 'I did want just one more holiday in the sun . . .'

It was the anniversary of his successful operation and the day before we were all to drive to Greece.

He died ten days later.

Supplementary reading

Books
Colling, Dr Aubrey (ed.). *Coronary Care in the Community* (1977): Croom Helm, London.

Croog, Sydney H. and Levine, Sol. *The Heart Patient Recovers: Social and Psychological Factors* (1977): Human Societies Press, New York and London.

Finlayson, Angela and McEwen, James. *Coronary Heart Disease and Patterns of Living* (1977): Croom Helm, London; Prodist, New York.

American Heart Association Cookbook (2nd ed.): American Heart Association, 53-001-A.

Other Publications
Heart Attack – Prevention and Treatment (a Family Doctor booklet): The British Medical Association.

Advice for those Recovering from a Heart Attack (pamphlet, 1978): Dr M.F. Oliver and Dr A.L. Muir, Scottish Health Education Unit, HMSO, Scotland.

What is Angina? (leaflet): Heart Research Series No. 4, British Heart Foundation, London.

Modern Heart Medicines (leaflet): Heart Research Series No. 6,

British Heart Foundation, London.

How to Control Your Weight and *The Facts about Cholesterol* (leaflet): Heart Research Series No. 7, British Heart Foundation, London.

Is It Blood Pressure? (leaflet): Heart Research Series No. 8, British Heart Foundation, London.

Reducing the Risk of a Coronary (leaflet, 1976): The Chest, Heart and Stroke Association, London, Edinburgh and Belfast.

Coronary After Care – general advice for the coronary patient (leaflet, 1975): The Chest and Heart Association, London, Edinburgh and Belfast.

*Heart Facts – 1979 (pamphlet): Annual publication by the American Heart Association, 55-005-C.

*Heart Attack (leaflet): American Heart Association, 51-010-B.

*Heart Attack – How to Reduce Your Risk (pamphlet): American Heart Association, 50-007-A.

Coronary Heart Disease: A New Zealand Report (1971): National Heart Foundation of New Zealand.

Diet and Coronary Heart Disease (1974): Report on Health and Social Subjects No. 7, Department of Health and Social Security, HMSO, London.

The Care of the Patient with Coronary Heart Disease (1975): Report of a Joint Working Party of the Royal College of Physicians of London and the British Cardiac Society, *Journal of the Royal College of Physicians,* Vol. 10, No. 1, October.

Prevention of Coronary Heart Disease (1976): Report of a Joint Working Party of the Royal College of Physicians of London and the British Cardiac Society, *Journal of the Royal College of Physicians,* Vol. 10, No. 3, April.

Services for Cardiovascular Emergencies (1975): Report of a World Health Organization Expert Committee, WHO, Geneva.

The Prevention of Coronary Heart Disease (1976): Report of a Working Group of the World Health Organization, WHO, Copenhagen.

Preventing Coronary Heart Disease (1978): European Society of Cardiology, Van Gorcum Assen, The Netherlands.

*These and many other publications are available from The American Heart Association.

Index

alcohol intake 67, 113–14
ambulance 76; cardiac 44, 76, 81–2; requesting 44
anastomosis 58
angina 41, 50, 111; symptoms of 56–7, 74
anxiety: after heart attack 91–2, 100; as a symptom 32; wives' 96, 101
arm, pain in 32, 34, 74
arteries, hardening of 54–6, 110–11
atheroma *see* arteries

bed rest 86–7, 101
blood 51–2; dilation of 57
blood pressure 52; high 66, 99, 115; low 54
breastbone, pain beneath 74
breathlessness 32, 39, 47, 75

chest pain 32, 72–3; in case studies of symptoms 11, 13, 20, 21, 24, 34, 35, 36
cholesterol 63–4, 67, 109
complexion 39
consciousness, diminished 32, 39

contraceptive pill 67
convalescence *see* recovery
coronary *see* heart attack

death, threat of 89
depression 91, 100
diabetics 66–7
diagnosis 22, 80; by patients' wives 38
diarrhoea 14
diet 8, 61–5, 109–14
dizziness 75
doctors 106; GPs consulted before attack 31; visits from 104
doctors' receptionists 12

electro-cardiogram (ECG) 31, 53, 80
emergency 11–27; telephone use in 36–7
emotional factors 68
enzymes in blood 80
exercise 8, 67, 105–6, 112, 113, 115

facial appearance 39, 75
faintness 32

INDEX

family 95, 103
fats (diet) 61–5, 99, 111
fibre, dietary 62–3, 67, 113
fibrillating heart 79–81
first aid 70–71

health: consciousness 68–9; neglect of 42
heart: anatomy of 51–2; blood supply to 53; function of 51–3; importance of, for self image 93; muscle 53, 54, 56, 86; scar 58, 86
heart attack 28–49; comparative incidence of 59–60, 99; coping with 75–8; fatal 61, 77–8; increase in deaths from 50, 55, 58–9; knowledge of 38; life after 89–107; patients put to bed 39–40
heartbeat 72
heaviness, feeling of 15, 21, 32, 57, 74

indigestion, feelings of 32–6 *passim*, 48, 77
infarct 57
insomnia 101
irritability 38, 42; after heart attack 100
ischaemic heart disease 50

lifestyle: guidance on 93, 104–5; sedentary 99
lipoproteins 63, 114

medical help, requesting 8, 18, 29, 37–8, 40–49
myocardial infarction *see* heart attack

neck, pain in 32

obesity 66, 113
occasional extrasystoles 72
oxygen shortage 75

pain 39, 47; relief 89 *see also specific parts of the body*
palpitations 71–2
patients: characteristics of 31, 61; general health of 31; self-concept 94–5; self-examination by 91–2
personality factors 39, 99–100
perspiration *see* sweating
polyunsaturated fats 62, 64, 112
prevention 108–15
pulse rate 54, 76

recovery 86–107; inactivity during 101; medical attitudes to 97
restlessness 32, 34, 39, 47
resuscitation, cardiac 70, 80

self-help groups 106–7
sexual activity 101, 102–3, 104
shoulders, pain in 32, 34, 74
sleep 38
smoking 8, 65–6, 99, 111, 114–15
stress 67–8, 98
stroke 55
stumbling 39
sweating 32, 39, 47–8; in studies of symptoms
symptoms 11–27, 74–6, recovery 103; typical holding 44–6

tightness in chest 74
tingling sensation 57
tiredness 31–2, 38
treatment 78–85; at home 17, 97, different types compared 82–4; in coronary care 79–80, 90; in hospital 17, 88, 97

vegetable oils 114
vomiting 13, 16, 24, 32, 39, 75

water, hard and soft 66
weakness 13
weight 66, 113, 114
wives and associates 99, 102-3; decision to call medical help 42-9, 71; effect of husband's attack on 95-6, 102-3; self-help groups for 106-7
women: examples of coping with emergencies Chapter 1 *passim*; heart attacks in 60, 73
work 67; overwork 98; returning to 105